ALZHEIMER'S:

A MESSAGE OF HOPE

Can it be Prevented?
Can it be Improved?
Can it be Reversed?

ALZHEIMER'S:

A MESSAGE OF HOPE

Can it be Prevented?
Can it be Improved?
Can it be Reversed?

Dr. Abraham Isaac Anbar

arbor books

For further information, please contact:

Arbor Books, Inc.
19 Spear Road, Suite 202
Ramsey, NJ 07446
877-822-2500

Book design:

ARBOR BOOKS, INC.
www.arborbooks.com

Printed in the United States

Alzheimer's:A Message of Hope
Dr. Abraham Isaac Anbar

1. Title 2. Author 3. Health/Medicine

Library of Congress Control Number: 2005938137

ISBN: 0-9771870-6-3

Table of Contents

ALZHEIMER'S:

A MESSAGE OF HOPE

Can it be…

Prevented?

Improved ?

Reversed?

Acknowledgements

This book is dedicated to all the patients whom I have cared for and who taught me through their pain and suffering that healthy living is the most precious gift we possess. Countless organizations and people over many years have been instrumental in supporting the vision, work and ideals of the Anbar Institute, including the Quebec Ministry of Health, Union leadership, and some extraordinary individuals.

Tina Nelson, whose endless support and exceptional intuitive management skills helped me to establish psychoneurological therapeutic institutes for patients afflicted with mental disorders and disabilities.

Mathilda Parise from the Gaspe peninsula of Quebec, who appeared as though out of nowhere, when I started the first Institute, and took over the care of patients with such an overwhelming flow of love, common sense and grit, helping so many patients to improve far beyond the expectations of the clinical staff.

Dr. Victorin Voyer of the University of Montreal, psychiatrist, psychoanalyst and above all an exceptionally giving person to all who knew him. His involvement in the Institute was invaluable.

Dr. John Howlett, professor of medicine at McGill University, and Medical Director of Saint Mary's Hospital in Montreal, who believed so fundamentally in our vision of addressing all aspects contributing to disease– from the physical and psychological to the spiritual, and who did everything in his power to support my work in making this vision a reality.

Dr. John Moore, Dean of the McGill University Graduate School of Social Work, who first invited me to be on the faculty as an Associate Professor of Psychiatry, and who understood my vision of what a therapeutic environment could and should be, and the healing effect it can have on the patients and their families. Dr. Moore did all he could to support and help me establish the first of the Anbar Institutes, while encouraging me to proceed with this vision and not be confined only to what currently existed in the medical community.

To my friend Joseph Pilates for his enthusiasm and involvement with us over the years in developing our therapeutic physical fitness programs in our institutions in Canada.

Yogi Vishnudevananda who as a young man contributed his belief and devotion to the formation of our health programs, and who subsequently went on to introduce Hatha yoga in Canada and the U.S., which today has become a staple at so many leading medical centers in the adjunctive treatment of chronic illnesses and stress related disorders.

To Antoine Pare, Queen's Council, who dedicated himself for over 50 years to the Anbar Institute as legal council and friend.

All of these people came to realize through their involvement with our work that the choice of a healthy lifestyle is a gift of nature that must be preemptively respected and continuously followed. Our health is our own responsibility and we must learn to assume it as early in life as possible if we wish to be healthy, free of sickness and to live fully and actively, as nature intended.

The purpose of this book is to share with the readers my own unique experiences, which have taught and guided me toward understanding the components of health, disease prevention and recovery.

The book is intended to be an educational tool to help people prevent Alzheimer's, as well as to help families of patients choose a direction of care that will benefit the victim and other family members. The book has no intent to criticize or offend any other existing ways of treatment. Sharing information from experiences and the resulting development of insight is the key to good education. To paraphrase an ancient Chinese proverb, "An intelligent person learns from his own experiences and mistakes. An ignorant person does not. A wise person learns from the experiences and mistakes of others." The patients were my best teachers. Let us all be wise and learn.

It is my hope that many of the readers will, in some way, benefit from this book. But even if only one person will, I shall consider my efforts to have been amply rewarded.

—*Dr. A. I. Anbar*
Chicago, Illinois
2005

Preface

I was blessed with having exceptional parents. Like most people, my understanding and respect for their wisdom grew as I began adulthood. My appreciation for their insights and foresights continues to increase, and I have come to realize that this evolution will never end.

My single most important objective has always been to impart their gift of life's lessons to my own family. Again, as for most of us, this is no easy task. But no worthwhile pursuit ever is.

My mother passed away prematurely from cancer. My father is now 83 years old, and is the picture of health. I cannot do anything to reclaim time and lost opportunities with my mother. It is too late. Like anyone who has suffered such a loss, there are regrets, but in retrospect, had she practiced a more healthy lifestyle herself, she would have been able to live longer, perhaps even avoiding sickness altogether.

I work in the senior housing industry. I witness, experience, and even feel the pain and suffering of scores of people. Is it part of the natural order to age with debilitating sickness and degenerative disease? Is it preordained somehow? Why do some people become sick but others do not? Why do some of the ill recover while others continue their downward spiral?

There are a myriad of questions, perplexities and challenges that confront us all. There is much confusion about health care issues, causes of disease, cures, drugs, political and financial interests. Whom should we listen to? Whom can we trust? Who has the answers? Are there any answers?

During the course of my life, I have watched as my father, Dr. A. I. Anbar, who has been involved in the health care field for over sixty years now, defied every norm and convention possible in his search for answers. In the field of healthcare, he has been an inspiration and a pioneer like no other. He repeatedly has seen truth before proof exists. His insights have never been limited to a particular agenda, lobby group or financial interest. His goal throughout his entire professional career has been to discover underlying causes, find solutions and share with others what he has learned.

He always created order from chaos, direction where there was none, and clarity of vision from obscurity.

In my own effort to provide answers to the many families I meet with who must face the challenge of caring for a loved one fallen ill, I have found myself offering the same answers as everyone else. But I wanted to do more. To this end, I asked my father to write a book that would offer his insights, provide hope to us all, and help contribute to the ultimate goal of discovering how to live in a world free of degenerative disease.

—*Dan Emmett Anbar*
Chicago, IL

Introduction

Nothing is so powerful as an idea whose time has come.
—Victor Hugo

For over 50 years, Dr. Anbar has been practicing the principles he describes in this book. They have formed the foundation for his development of various healthcare projects, from establishing the largest private healthcare organization in Canada to developing the world's largest medical diagnostic, early detection and treatment complex, which treats 55,000 patients a month. Over the years, his vision has remained the same, but its application to healthcare has grown.

Today, Dr. Anbar's approach toward improving and reversing illnesses, such as cardiovascular disease and dementia, has been validated in laboratories and clinical practice, and is recognized as the cutting-edge of healthcare. It has been adopted by the federal and state governments in various contexts, from workers' compensation to the national health initiative Healthy People 2010. But in the early years this was not the case.

It has always been my father's steadfast conviction that the fundamental principles of nature hold true, and that people can practice these principles as part of their lifestyle. Proper diet, healthy beliefs and interactions, and exercise are effective in living healthy lives and overcoming illness.

One of the principles I heard as a child was that the body could inherently heal itself if we understood how to help it. Along those lines, my family consumed quantities of raw fruits and vegetables in addition to nuts and grains. But to most people in the 1940's and 50's, and particularly the medical establishment, the notion that food could be used to prevent illness was often seen as preposterous and "not medically sound."

It wasn't always easy growing up with parents whose views on health and nutrition were so disparate from those of my friends' families. While Dad worked to promote his vision of healthcare, Mom struggled on the home front to raise her kids according to these principles. This was at a time when not eating meat and limiting sugar, white flower and milk products seemed like heresy. My parents also engaged us in "strange" fitness practices, with the likes of Joseph Pilates and Moshe Feldenkrais, and dragged us to Swami Vishnudevananda's yoga studio.

When other children were consuming a more conventional diet of macaroni and cheese, hot dogs and white bread (which was touted as helping kids "grow in 12 different ways"), potato chips and soda, my siblings and I ate snacks of fresh fruits, vegetables and nuts. This didn't always seem fair, especially when advertisements on TV showed how much fun the other kids were having with their food. But our parents prevailed, and we gradually understood the connection between lifestyle and health.

As I grew, I began to see how encompassing my father's beliefs actually were. I remember, when I visited his residential Institutes for children, how I was struck by its positive atmosphere: kids were running, laughing and playing, surrounded by loving adults who gave of themselves unconditionally. Everyone seemed to be happier than in the outside world. When I visited seniors living in the healthcare resort my father established to replace the prevalent "nursing home" model, I knew these were very special places which made people feel happier. Healthier. Better. And I was profoundly moved by what I saw.

Years later, I more fully grasped the concepts in practice at the Anbar Institute, such as the impact of a therapeutic community, and multidisciplinary treatment for chronic and degenerative illnesses. These approaches got to the root of a problem, rather than focusing primarily on symptoms. I saw the importance of empowering patients, educating and supporting them through the recovery process. I had witnessed how the body could heal itself and how people who were ill could get better. Everyone, from a psychotic child to a depressed, arthritic senior, could improve when given the opportunity.

My father has always believed that improvement is possible despite the odds. This conviction reflects his own experiences growing up during the British Mandate in Palestine through the birth of Israel. And when he began his education and career in America, his "can do" spirit was very much in synch with the unique era of the late 1940's and 50's.

To understand, in part, what gave rise to my father's attitude that "anything is possible if you set your mind to it" requires a brief glimpse into the cultural attitude of the time.

America in the 1950's was a place of idealism and heroism. When World War II ended, veterans returned to create new lives for themselves. The GI Bill provided them with college or vocational education, as well as one year of unemployment compensation. It also provided loans to buy homes and start businesses. At that time, millions of people were able to own their own homes, turning the American Dream into reality.

The post-war era marked a period of unprecedented energy and the birth of the civil rights movement. It was an era characterized by space travel and a sense that nothing was impossible.

It was against this backdrop that developments were also unfolding in healthcare. This progress gave rise to the concept of the therapeutic community, based upon the philosophy that many forms of mental illness are treatable with a combination of psychoanalysis and occupational therapy. This was a profoundly important contribution to healthcare which would resurface in the 1990's, but its antecedents can be found in pedagogy, therapeutic education, social medicine and the changing human relations that took place between the two great European wars.

It was a period when our system of healthcare valued life regardless of cost and saw human interaction as one of the most powerful tools in the healing process.

The therapeutic community movement, which grew out of this period in time, holds a multidisciplinary view of health drawn from many different principles—including analytic, behavourial, creative, educational and humanistic-combined with the best conventional medical practices.

In addition to staff physicians and psychologists, the therapeutic community included teachers, art and occupational therapists, physical therapists and therapeutic fitness instructors (influenced by the work of my childhood friends Pilates, Feldenkrais and Vishnudevananda). One's own belief system also played a large role, so clergy were part of the staffing. This multidisciplinary model, employed by Dr. Anbar since the early 1950's, served to address the multifaceted roots of illness and to ultimately find what was needed for rehabilitation.

Fundamental to the therapeutic communities of the Anbar Institutes were the concepts that everyone-children, adolescents, seniors with neurological problems, or individuals suffering from alcohol/substance abuse could improve and that by doing (and eating) the right thing, people do better.

But these beliefs weren't shared by all. My father told me of a government health inspector who came to the Institute and wanted to know why the wheat flour used to bake the bread and the sugar in the kitchen were dirty. He had never heard of whole wheat or brown sugar before! And, despite their beliefs, the Anbar Institute was forced to serve milk because it was required by the government and expected by parents.

By 1992, things had begun to change considerably. Dr. Spock was alerting parents to potential health risks of milk products. Studies had linked anemia and childhood-onset diabetes to milk exposure in infancy. Dr. Neal Barnard, President of Physicians Committee for Responsible Medicine, discussed how dairy proteins could destroy the insulin-producing cells of the pancreas. Researchers found that breast-fed children were largely protected against diabetes, compared to those fed cows' milk formulas.

In 1994, the American Academy of Pediatrics reported that more than 90 studies were concerned about milk's link to diabetes. In 1996, the Dietary Guidelines for Americans, the nation's blueprint for all nutrition programs, was rewritten to officially acknowledge the benefits of vegetarian diets. By 1998, more than 50 million copies of Dr. Spock's book-encouraging proper diets to beat the odds of two out of three children later developing heart disease or cancer were sold, making it second in sales only to the Bible.

Milk, Cholesterol, Cardiovascular Disease and Alzheimer's

Milk consumption is related to arteriosclerosis (hardening of the arteries). Data from the Framingham Study show that cholesterol levels measured in young adults are predictive of death, due to coronary heart disease (CHD), 30 years later.

Epidemiologic data support the relationship between childhood and adult cholesterol levels, and show a relationship between high cholesterol in the children and premature CHD in the parents. Pathologic findings have provided further evidence of the early development of atherosclerosis: young U.S. soldiers killed in the Korean War were found, with high frequency, to have advanced coronary artery lesions. In fact, the arteries of the young Americans were similar to those of the 60-year old Koreans who did not consume milk.

More recently, a team from Newcastle University has discovered that elderly people who suffer from heart disease may also be at risk of Alzheimer's disease. They found that almost 80% of the patients in their study with Alzheimer's disease also had arteriosclerosis, further implying a relationship between diet, heart disease and Alzheimer's.

The 1995 publication of the Dietary Guidelines for Americans, produced by the U.S. Department of Agriculture and the Department of Human Services, notes that: Diet is important to health at all stages of life.

Many genetic, environmental, behavioral, and cultural factors can affect health. Understanding family history of disease or risk factors-body weight and fat distribution, blood pressure, and blood cholesterol, for example-can help people make more informed decisions about actions that can improve health prospects. Food choices are among the most pleasurable and effective of these actions.

Healthful diets help children grow, develop, and do well in school. They enable people of all ages to work productively and feel their best. Food choices also can help to reduce the risk for chronic diseases, such as heart disease, certain cancers, diabetes, stroke, and osteoporosis, that are leading causes of death and disability among Americans. Good diets can reduce major risk factors for chronic diseases-factors such as obesity, high blood pressure, and high blood cholesterol.

In 2000, a USDA study showed how plant sterols lower cholesterol. Today plant sterols are being added to orange juice and sold as a guaranteed way to lower cholesterol. Unfortunately, for most people, it is easier to buy the orange juice than to add the raw vegetables to their diet-which, in fact, would do much more to prevent and repair damage to the body.

Since the mid-80's, research published in the Journal of the American Medical Association and the New England Journal of Medicine has demonstrated how vegetarian diets, stress reduction and group support is the only method for reversing heart disease, the number one cause of death in the U.S., without the use of drugs or surgery.

In 2003, The National Cancer Institute-FDA launched an initiative in which stickers affixed to bananas read, "Diets rich in fruits and vegetables may reduce the risk of some types of cancers and other chronic diseases."

What was radical or even eccentric in the 1950's has now become the cutting-edge in medicine

Vegetarian and Vegan Diets

The following recommendations and summary of research was prepared by the Nutrition Panel of the Physicians Committee for Responsible Medicine.

Increasingly, vegetables, grains, fruits, legumes, and nuts are proving to be the optimal foods for children. Rich in complex carbohydrates, protein, fiber, vitamins, and minerals, they form the foundation for dietary habits that support a lifetime of health. Research indicates that adults who consume fruits and vegetables are those who consumed these foods during childhood. The following are some of the long-term advantages of plant-based diets:

- The prevalence of hypertension among vegetarians is about one-third to one-half that of non-vegetarians. A study of Caucasian Seventh-day Adventists found hypertension in 22 percent of omnivores, but only 7 percent of vegetarians. Among African-Americans, the prevalence was 44 percent of omnivores and 18 percent of vegetarians. Adopting a vegetarian diet significantly lowers blood pressure in both normal and hypertensive individuals.

- Cholesterol levels are much lower in vegetarians. Vegetarian diets reduce serum cholesterol levels to a much greater degree than is achieved with the National Cholesterol Education Program Step Two diet. In one study published in The Lancet, total cholesterol in those following a vegetarian diet for 12 months decreased by 24.3 percent.

- Cancer rates for vegetarians are 25 to 50 percent below population averages, even after controlling for smoking, body mass index, and socioeconomic status. One study found that people who include generous amounts of fruits and vegetables in their daily diets have lower rates of cancers of the lung, breast, colon, bladder, stomach, mouth, larynx, esophagus, pancreas, and cervix compared to people who avoid such foods.

- Obesity is a major contributor to many serious illnesses, and is much less common among vegetarians, compared to the general population. Vegetarians are, on average, about 10 percent leaner than omnivores.

- Plant-based diets may encourage a later menarche, which has been shown to be associated with reduced risk of breast cancer in epidemiologic studies.

- Fruits and vegetables contain antioxidant substances, such as vitamin C, vitamin E, and carotenoids, which protect cells against oxidative damage, which is related to cancer risk and other health problems. The multitude of phytochemicals found in various fruits, vegetables, grains, legumes, and nuts are thought to protect against heart disease and cancer.

Psychosocial Support and Therapy

The importance of the psychosocial aspects of life, both in contributing to illness and in their effectiveness in prevention and intervention, was documented in Lancet in 1989. Research conducted by Dr. David Spiegel demonstrated how women with breast cancer who participated in supportive-expressive group therapy lived twice as long as women who were not in group therapy.

The effectiveness of group therapy and therapeutic environments has a long-standing history, which has become part of popular culture.

The book and motion picture *I Never Promised You a Rose Garden* depicted Joanne Greenberg's experience at Chestnut Lodge Hospital in Rockville, Maryland, during which she was in psychoanalytic treatment with Frieda Fromm-Reichmann. It was important to note to what extent even certain types of schizophrenias could be healed with proper interpersonal support and therapy.

The model of a therapeutic community as described in this book dates back to 1954 at the Anbar Institute, when the modalities employed went far beyond psychological intervention to include nutrition, therapeutic cognitive and physical exercise, and other essential components.

I saw how a therapeutic community could have the same effect and warmth as a parent's love. Its environment and encouragement reminded me of my father's refrain: "By overcoming your fears, you become stronger. By doing, rather than just wishing, you move forward and improve. It is in the doing that you grow and achieve." Today social scientists have defined these characteristics in terms of positive psychology and clinical efficacy, attributes which are fundamental in improving chronic health conditions.

Healing is a Broad Concept

The treatment approach described in this book-systematically preventing, improving and reversing many chronic and debilitating health conditions-has come to be known by various terms, and is practiced in many different ways with varying degrees of success. The general approach is referred to as mind/body, behavioral, biopsychosocial or interdisciplinary medicine. Whatever the name, it is a scientific approach proven to reverse cardiovascular disease, chronic pain, insomnia and irritable bowel syndrome, often without surgery or drugs.

Behavioral medicine is an interdisciplinary field concerned with the development and integration of biomedical, sociocultural, psychosocial, and behavioral knowledge relevant to health and illness, and the application of this knowledge to disease prevention, health promotion, etiology, diagnosis, treatment and rehabilitation.

As initially practiced at the Anbar Institute in Quebec, Canada, beginning in 1954, the focus of treatment involved an interdisciplinary team to educate patients on improving their condition and becoming more involved in taking care of themselves. Twenty-three years later, a conference at Yale University further defined the interdisciplinary field of behavioral medicine.

Because of the effectiveness of mind/body medicine, testimony before the U.S Senate led to the National Institutes of Health establishing mind/body medical institutes in the U.S.

In April of 2005, the California Legislature joined other states in passing regulation which incorporated the multidisciplinary approach as the treatment of choice for chronic pain within the workers' compensation system.

Increasingly, this approach is being scientifically-validated as the treatment of choice for Alzheimer's and related dementias because it represents the most comprehensive intervention for prevention, treatment and rehabilitation.

The principles outlined in this approach are aligned with the goals of the U.S. government initiative Healthy People 2010 "to help individuals of all ages increase life expectancy and improve their quality of life."

Those engaged in these practices are experiencing one of the most important frontiers of healthcare, in which lifestyle and belief systems are recognized as core to prevention and rehabilitation. Mind/body medicine and the multidisciplinary treatment of illness are both life-altering and life-affirming.

I invite you to discover the power of what healthy living can achieve for you or a loved one. You will be glad you did.

Tomer Anbar, Ph.D., CGP, CTC
San Diego, CA
March 2006

Foreword

I am Pain...
This is then the truth I bring you,
That I hurt you, but to warn you,
Not to harm you, but to heal you,
That I come to guide and teach you.

I am God's most blessed angel!
Sent to point the way to virtue,
Sent to teach the noblest manhood,
Sent to rouse the Soul to Action!

—C.J. Buell
Excerpt from *Pain's Soliloquy*

There she stands, bent over, a faraway look in her eyes, the woman who cared for you when you were ill, who taught you to read, to cook, to sing, to look both ways before crossing the street. She is your mother.

But these days you must read her mail, because for her the words and letters are a meaningless jumble. You must also prepare her meals, because she might leave the stove unattended again and the oven or burners on; last week the house nearly burned down when an overheated frying pan caught fire.

You must also act as her eyes and guide her everywhere; the last time she went out alone she became lost and disoriented. On bad days, she lashes out and abuses you in anger. On good days, she simply does not know who you are. For she is suffering from Alzheimer's disease.

If pain is a messenger, to whom does it speak? In the case of Alzheimer's, it speaks to all of us, the healthy and the sick alike, and it has much to tell.

This is a book about understanding and unlocking the secret messages of Alzheimer's, the most emotionally painful of the degenerative illnesses. It is about transcending its pain and suffering, and about renewal and recovery. My purpose is to heighten awareness of the fact that becoming ill, not only with Alzheimer's but with a host of chronic and debilitating diseases, is in large measure a result of personal choice, out of ignorance or by default, and not simply a tragic bolt from the blue. That is the bad news. The good news is that we hold in our hands the power of healing: we can actually preempt and, in many cases, even reverse Alzheimer's, and I will explain ways of doing so. Quite simply, our health and the quality and duration of our lives depend on the lifestyle choices we make. It is destructive living and unhealthy lifestyles that are the primary factors in causing sickness, not, as we usually assume, bacteria or viruses that invade and ruin our body. They are only the result of the weakness and not its cause. They are able to damage us because we have become enfeebled by poor diet, sedentary living, and cognitive, emotional, psychological, interpersonal and spiritual instability which, as medical science is discovering, contribute to severely decreasing our immunity and making us vulnerable to so many chronic illnesses, including depression and anxiety. Unfortunately, medical science has largely defined symptoms as disease, and emphasis has been wrongly placed on primarily removing symptoms. Even though in this way messengers of pain may be temporarily silenced, we continue to become ill and to die before our time.

Medical pharmacology continually produces stronger and stronger drugs with which to combat disease, yet messengers of pain and illness continue arriving uninterruptedly. In terms of percentages as well as actual numbers, more people have cancer, heart disease, arthritis, and Alzheimer's than ever before. However, neither science nor medicine is able to save us from ourselves; medicine cannot make us eat a clean, nutritious diet rich in antioxidants, nor can it provide emotional and psychological supports to ward off deadly stress; it cannot invent a pill which forces us to exercise. We know we should, yet far too many find it impossible to commit to the simplest exercise plan, such as daily walking. And yet nutritious diet, regular exercise and stress reduction are the strongest weapons we have for repelling or recovering from Alzheimer's and other diseases.

For those already sick, it is often impossible to summon the strength to change behaviors that cause sickness in the first place. The task is daunting even for healthy individuals. So the vast majority takes the path of least resistance and persists with harmful habits usually acquired at a young age—diets of poor nutritional value or, worse, junk food coupled with sedentary activities such as excessive television, which too often reinforces distorted beliefs promoted by negative financial interests. These are harsh realities that no medicine or drug can alter.

In fact, the pervasiveness of drugs in our culture—with prescriptions raining down on us for everything from headaches to irritable bowel—contributes to attitudes of passivity and helplessness regarding our health. We believe that all we need do is visit the doctor, swallow Mother's Little Helper, and watch vim, vigor, and vitality instantly return. But things haven't quite worked out that way.

It is important to bear in mind that medical science can

only discover that which exists. For example, body toxins were at work destroying immunity, and phytonutrients were strengthening immunity, long before science recognized their existence and gave those names. Slowly but surely science is beginning to grasp principles of nature that have been understood and put into practice by certain individuals and communities throughout history. References to such practices can be found in the ancient literature of many cultures. Hippocrates, the father of Western medicine, declared over two and a half millennia ago that "food is our medicine."

In the contemporary world, we can witness the results of lives lived according to natural principles, such as among the Hunza, who thrive atop the "roof of the world," the mountainous region adjoining Afghanistan and Tibet where diseases like Alzheimer's are totally unknown. Later on, we will review the Hunza lifestyle in some detail, for it teaches important lessons and presents a fascinating model we would do well to emulate in certain aspects.

We are all a part of our environment, emotionally as well as physically, and in these pages we will examine a number of environmental factors that bear directly on Alzheimer's. It is a good bet that if our environment is healthy, we, too, will be healthy. If not, we are most likely to fall sick. And the only way to permanently solve any health problem is to remove its cause and strengthen the body through natural, wholesome living.

However, once sickness has struck, the best cure is to immerse the sufferer in a therapeutic environment that provides healthy living, and excludes everything unhealthy. Where food is natural and abundant in nutrients; where air and water are uncontaminated; where physical and mental activity are plentiful; where stress resilience is developed; where people actually connect with each other; where spiritual opportunities exist, and where the devastating effects of

Alzheimer's can be slowed, improved or even reversed. The reader may well ask: does such an Eden exist? In this book I will describe some of the treatments, activities, and case histories which occurred during my career, before my very eyes.

Unlike some nursing homes that can very often be little more than "cemeteries-in-waiting," our therapeutic environments have brought about remarkable improvements in treating those with dementia, among many other ailments, and offers true hope to patients and families. Wonderful results have happened for some; I believe therefore they can happen for many. It is my deep desire, my dream, and my firm belief that with a comprehensive approach to healing through the creation of truly therapeutic environments, our hope can become a reality.

As an example, when Alzheimer's patients begin *helping one another to improve*, they stimulate and encourage each other to a far greater degree than any staff member could, because it is emotionally important for those with common health problems to seek common solutions. Self-sharing and communication are powerful healing instruments.

Years ago, when I established therapeutic institutions for children with mental disorders and disabilities, I saw that those who began helping others were the first to improve. Their insight into the fears and hopes of their peers was amazingly telling. Doctors and nurses received as much uplift from these children as the children did from them.

One of the saddest aspects confronting Alzheimer's patients and their families is that the disease robs them of what should be the best phase of life, their seniority. Like flowers, men and women should be at their richest and most beautiful in this most developed phase of the life cycle.

A human being, wrote the well known scholar/psychologist Carl Jung, would not live to be seventy or eighty or more if longevity were meaningless. The last part of life must therefore possess its own significance and be something greater than a mere afterthought to one's youth. Could it be, he asked, that gaining wisdom and a contemplation of the spiritual are the purpose of the latter half of life? If this is true, then it is imperative that we prevent and reverse Alzheimer's disease so that all may achieve full human potential; so we will not have to witness any of our mothers' or fathers' agonizing descents into dementia. *We can accomplish this by paying close attention to first principles of health,* which is this book's theme. Herein lies our true hope and great opportunity. There is no point in anybody trying to invent new principles, since we need only recall what has long been known: healthy attitudes, the eating of nutrient-rich fruits, vegetables, nuts, legumes, and elimination or at least reduction of meats consumed, and the elimination of processed, chemically-laced, high-fat/high-sugar foods, along with regular exercise, will surely make for healthier minds and bodies. Not only can we hope, but we can choose, to lead lives in the full bloom of health until the end of our natural life span, which science today indicates can run to 120 years. In the natural world, flowers sprout, grow, and die because it is time. The same is true of animals. Only human beings are struck down prematurely, for only human beings make self-destructive choices.

Nature's message, then, is that instead of expecting disease we should choose to live disease-free lives. The ability to choose—the inherent human gift—enables us to be proactive rather than reactive. We will know that we have chosen wisely when we no longer receive messages of pain and suffering, but regular bodily reports of robust health and vigor.

Chapter One

What Is Alzheimer's?

Alzheimer's disease n. a degenerative disorder that affects the
brain and causes dementia, especially later in life.
—Microsoft Encarta College Dictionary

Reference books can define this disease in such a few words, but
what is this affliction that levels presidents and grandmothers
alike? Why does it seem that we are hearing more and more
about it, either from news reports or personal acquaintances?

The perception that the incidence of Alzheimer's is growing is a valid one. The Alzheimer's Association has predicted
that the number of people suffering from Alzheimer's in the
United States will increase by an alarming 350 percent within
the first fifty years of this century. The Association estimates
that there were about five million Alzheimer's sufferers in the
country as the century began and it predicts that, by the year
2050, that number will have climbed to 14 million. Some estimates are even higher.

So, who wants to talk about Alzheimer's? Not any healthy person, certainly. Not any child of a beloved aging parent. In the natural order of things, the parent will die first, and that is a thought most of us resolutely keep at bay in order to enjoy the time we have together.

However, it is impossible to escape the reality as we watch the aging process line our parents' faces, slow their step, and confuse their minds. It is this last ravage that is the most difficult to bear, especially when we see ourselves being erased from our parents' memory and find ourselves helpless to stop it.

There are many conditions that affect the aging mind, but none may be as heartbreaking as Alzheimer's. Its effects are so horrific that our minds instinctively recoil from the thought of it, but its seriousness and pervasiveness require that we face it head on in order to combat it.

And there are global implications as well. The World Health Organization (WHO) estimated that of the 37 million people around the world who had dementia in the year 2000, a substantial majority had Alzheimer's. When the forecast for the disease's growth in the United States is interpolated for the world's sufferers, the resulting prognosis is staggering.

Approximately 50 percent of us will develop Alzheimer's if we live past the age of eighty-five, and of all deaths caused by dementia, seventy percent are related to Alzheimer's. A small group, about 10 percent, of those who develop Alzheimer's will do so before the age of 60. Their condition is known as early-onset familial Alzheimer's disease and is currently considered to be caused by an inherited genetic mutation.

Health officials estimate that an additional 20 million people are directly affected by Alzheimer's, although they do not suffer from the disease. These are the family members and caregivers, whose lives come to center around the disease as its symptoms worsen and the need for care intensifies.

The cost is measurable: more than $100 *billion* per year to treat Alzheimer's in the United States alone. And the price of the community's loss of the wealth of wisdom, experience, and leadership stolen by this disease, is incalculable. The victims' inability to live fully and gracefully their ripest years, as nature intended, is among the greatest of human tragedies.

In our culture, we have taken for granted that aging people are fragile, often sick, and are degenerating. Even the word "longevity," in our culture, connotes an extended life of extreme frailty and a deteriorating state of health and physicality.

Yet we know that people's lives can be transformed if they live under the right circumstances and conditions and live in a nurturing environment. Human beings are remarkably adaptive and resilient creatures; they can preempt and even recover from all sorts of degenerative conditions and disorders, and go on to lead healthy, productive, meaningful, and enjoyable lives, well past 100 years.

Alzheimer's never exists in a vacuum. Family history, medical history, nutritional status, environment, lifestyle, maturity, age and longevity are all related and play a role in its origin. It is unfortunate but highly telling that in our Western culture we perceive sickness as caused by bad luck or accident and equate age with infirmity, while viewing robust longevity as a fluke, a kind of winning lottery ticket printed from the genes of our ancestors. This attitude says much about our current state of health.

However, it is possible for people to be continuously well.

And so what is Alzheimer's and what is it not? Here are some definitions:

Alzheimer's

Is	Is Not
a chronic, degenerative disease	mental illness
Fatal	Unavoidable
a disease that affects older individuals	caused by aging
Treatable	Inevitable
a cause of dementia	the prevalent cause of memory loss
caused by a variety of factors	widely inherited
detectable with testing	apparent physically in its earliest stages

Quite often, the first symptom to appear is memory loss, which early on may be thought of as a normal occurrence in a world characterized by fast-paced schedules and sensory overload. As memory loss accelerates, however, family and friends, as well as the Alzheimer's sufferer, recognize it as a symptom of something gone horribly wrong. Traditionally, all anyone could do was watch helplessly as the disease worked its inexorable way through progressively debilitating stages.

While the degeneration is continuous, different groups of cells are damaged in turn, and the disease can be tracked as it moves from one stage to the next and the patient begins losing distinct abilities. Each sufferer's experience is somewhat unique; not all people experience all symptoms, nor do they experience them in the same order or with the same intensity during the progression of the disease.

The Alzheimer's Association notes that while experts can track the disease in a general way, any attempt at separating its stages involves artificial, arbitrary demarcation lines, given the rapidly changing nature of the disease. The Association's use of a seven-stage framework, available on its Internet home page, is based on a system developed by Barry Reisberg, M.D., clinical director of the New York University School of Medicine's Silberstein Aging and Dementia Research Center. The framework, which follows, corresponds to widely used concepts of mild, moderate, moderately severe, and severe Alzheimer's. It also notes which stages fall within the more general divisions of early-stage, mid-stage, and late-stage categories:

Stage 1: No Cognitive Impairment

Unimpaired individuals experience no memory problems; none are evident to a health care professional during medical interview.

Stage 2: Very Mild Decline

Individuals at this stage feel as if they have memory lapses, especially in forgetting familiar words or names or the location of keys, eyeglasses, or other everyday objects; yet these problems are not evident during a medical examination or apparent to friends, family, or co-workers.

Stage 3: Mild Cognitive Decline

Early-stage Alzheimer's can be diagnosed in some, but not all, individuals with these symptoms:

Friends, family, or co-workers begin to notice deficiencies. Problems with memory or concentration may be measurable in clinical testing or discernible during a detailed medical interview. Common difficulties include:

- Word or name-finding problems noticeable to family or close associates.
- Decreased ability to remember names when introduced to new people.

- Performance issues in social or work settings noticeable to family, friends, or co-workers.
- Reading a passage and retaining little material.
- Losing or misplacing a valuable object.
- Decline in ability to plan or organize.

Stage 4: Moderate Cognitive Decline

(Mild or early-stage Alzheimer's disease)

At this stage, a careful medical interview detects clear-cut deficiencies in the following areas:

- Decreased knowledge of recent events.
- Impaired ability to perform challenging mental arithmetic—for example, to count backward from 100 by 7s.
- Decreased capacity to perform complex tasks, such as marketing, planning dinner for guests, or paying bills and managing finances.
- Reduced memory of personal history.
- The affected individual may seem subdued and withdrawn, especially in socially or mentally challenging situations.

Stage 5: Moderately Severe Cognitive Decline

(Moderate or mid-stage Alzheimer's disease)

Major gaps in memory and deficits in cognitive function emerge. Some assistance with day-to-day activities becomes essential. At this stage, individuals may:

- Be unable during a medical interview to recall such important details as their current address, their telephone number, or the name of the college or high school from which they graduated.

- Become confused about where they are or about the date, day of the week, or season.

- Have trouble with less challenging mental arithmetic; for example, counting backward from 40 by 4s or from 20 by 2s.

- Need help choosing proper clothing for the season or occasion.

- Usually retain substantial knowledge about themselves and know their own name and the names of their spouse or children.

- Usually require no assistance with eating or using the toilet.

Stage 6: Severe Cognitive Decline

(Moderately severe or mid-stage Alzheimer's disease)

Memory difficulties continue to worsen, significant personality changes may emerge, and affected individuals need extensive help with daily activities. At this stage, individuals may:

- Lose most awareness of recent experiences and events as well as their surroundings.

- Recollect their personal history imperfectly, although they generally recall their own name.

- Occasionally forget the name of their spouse or primary caregiver but generally can distinguish familiar from unfamiliar faces.

- Need help getting dressed properly; without

supervision, may make such errors as putting pajamas over daytime clothes or shoes on wrong feet.

- Experience disruption of their normal sleep/waking cycle.

- Need help with handling details of toileting (flushing toilet, wiping and disposing of tissue properly).

- Have increasing episodes of urinary or fecal incontinence.

- Experience significant personality changes and behavioral symptoms, including suspiciousness and delusions (for example, believing that their caregiver is an imposter); hallucinations (seeing or hearing things that are not really there); or compulsive, repetitive behaviors such as hand wringing, or tissue shredding.

- Tend to wander and become lost.

Stage 7: Very Severe Cognitive Decline

(Severe or late-stage Alzheimer's disease)

This is the final stage when individuals lose ability to respond to their environment, the ability to speak, and ultimately, the ability to control movement.

- Frequently, individuals lose the capacity for recognizable speech, although words or phrases may occasionally be uttered.

- Individuals need help with eating and toileting, and there is general urinary incontinence.

- Individuals lose the ability to walk without assistance, and then the ability to sit without support, the ability to smile, and the ability to hold up their head. Reflexes become abnormal and muscles grow rigid. Swallowing is impaired.

Historically, Alzheimer's could only be definitely diagnosed through autopsy. Progress has been made, and tests are available that can differentiate Alzheimer's from other masking or mimicking dementias.

It may seem simplistic to note that in order for testing to occur, the individual must be aware that there is a problem. However, Alzheimer's can do extensive damage before any first or second-stage symptoms appear; therefore, individual awareness of warning signs is key to early detection.

Among the flags that may signal to the individual or family and friends that further testing is warranted are loss of hearing and of the sense of smell. These problems can be caused by other factors such as injury or chronic sinus infection. Once these causes are ruled out, it is time to consider that the problems are symptoms of disruption of neural function, or nerve damage. These nerves are among those affected the earliest by Alzheimer's.

Depression is also among the earliest signs that Alzheimer's might be present. The family member who loses his or her appetite for both food and life activities, has crying spells, or is constantly tired with no physical reason may be suffering from depression brought on by Alzheimer's.

Another symptom a nonprofessional may notice is the loss of spatial perception. A simple game is an easy home test for this symptom: place several objects on a table and have the individual look at them for one minute. Then, have him look away and recall what objects were present. Have friends or family members do the same as a control group. If the individual's score is much lower than the others, there could be concern that Alzheimer's is present (Cohen 1999).

When home tests and observations signal a problem, the next step is to follow up with professional diagnostic methods, including neuropsychological evaluations, EEG, CT scans, MRI, and serum chemistries. Alzheimer's can be misdiagnosed for other disorders, such as hypothyroidism, hypoglycemia, drug reactions, and others, so it is important that the complete physical include psychological and mental evaluation (Picoulin 2002).

Even with these procedures, misdiagnosis is possible. Experts in the field have developed what is considered to be the most accurate diagnostic tool by establishing criteria to be followed in the testing process. Working together to develop the criteria were the Alzheimer's Disease Related Disorders Association and the National Institute of Neurological and Communicative Disorders (ADRDA-NINCDS).

The Alzheimer's Association reports that misclassification and misdiagnosis for dementia and Alzheimer's was more than 30 percent before the use of the ADRDA-NINCDS testing process. That rate has fallen to below 5 percent with the testing, according to the Association.

The process has been augmented with two other tools, the NIA/AMA (National Institute on Aging/American Medical Association) and the DSM-III (Diagnostic and Statistical Manual of Mental Disorders—Fourth Edition). All three procedures render a positive diagnosis for Alzheimer's only if loss of intellectual abilities and impairment in memory are present. Additionally, a personality change or diminished language skills are also required for a positive diagnosis from NIA/AMA and DSM-III testing.

These symptoms are only half the picture of the devastation the body is undergoing. Unseen, nerves and synapses deteriorate and the body's complex communication network breaks down. This network's job is to process information about both the workings of the body and the world outside it, interpret, mediate, and trigger the bodily response.

The basic driver of this system is the neuron, the nerve cell, which receives signals and sends signals to other, differentiated neurons. In order to signal, the nerve cell manufactures neurotransmitters, chemical transmitter molecules, which it sends across the gap between it and the other nerve cell. The gap is the synapse.

Scientists have identified eight different neurotransmitters. They have also discovered a number of neuropeptide molecules, which regulate the effects of neurotransmitters.

In the healthy brain, signaling between neurons is rapid and completed with precision, aided in part by receptor molecules which recognize and bind specific neurotransmitters. Some nerves do not have receptors in their synapses, and they communicate by electrical transmission.

The brains of Alzheimer's patients lose neurons. As the disease progresses, this loss becomes severe enough to be measured, both in decreased size and weight of the brain. There is also a corresponding decrease in the chemical levels of neurotransmitters. These include acetylcholine, norepinephrine, and serotonin and their corresponding neuropeptide molecules.

Also characteristic of the brain of an Alzheimer's patient are lesions found in the cerebral cortex. These are neuritic plaques, deposits of neuron fragments surrounding a core of amyloid *b*-protein, and neurofibrillary tangles, twisted fibers of the protein *tau* with neurons.

So how does this process begin? Why do the nerve cells deteriorate? The answer may surprise you, because despite the fact that the majority of its victims are over the age of 60, Alzheimer's is not caused by age. If it were, the disease would appear in all humans once they passed the triggering age, much the same way permanent teeth or secondary sex charac-teristics make their appearance at their appointed moment.

Make no mistake about it; Alzheimer's is a disease as int-rusive and contrary to the normal processes of human biology as is the flu. It is *not* a byproduct of aging.

Sickness is always the result of causes and reasons. If we "catch" an infectious disease, the cause is attributed to parasitic bacteria or viruses that enter and infest our bodies. However, the real reason they can do so is because our immunity is low. If our immune system is properly functioning, those parasites cannot successfully invade our bodies, because our antibodies will destroy them.

The same is true of "free radicals" that we develop within our own bodies. Free radicals can cause degenerative disease and kill us, but only if our immunity is low. Free radicals are a natural byproduct of chemical reactions inside cells. Free radicals are oxy-gen molecules that lack one of their customary two electrons on the surface. To achieve stability, free radical oxygen molecules take an electron from a nearby molecule. They may attach them-selves to molecules on the surface of cells or even in the DNA of those cells (Fotuhi 2003).

A surface attack by free radicals causes holes, or pores, that allow water to escape from cells. Once dehydrated, cells can-not function efficiently and are susceptible to injury and death. The process is akin to the effect of rust on an unpro-tected surface. "Rust" away enough brain cells, and the con-dition of Alzheimer's has its foothold.

The cell's ability to produce new proteins is impaired when the free radical attack is on the DNA, and not the surface, of the cell. While day-to-day living causes some low-level damage to DNA that can be repaired, the sheer number of free radicals involved in an assault is overwhelming, and the DNA cannot repair itself.

Ironically, once free radicals begin inflicting damage, our bodies, in an attempt to compensate and restore equilibrium, cause further damage to the brain. Consider how an extremity of your body, your ankle or knee for example, will swell when sprained. The swelling is a protective measure taken by the body, indicating that immune cells have been rushed to the site to begin the task of cleaning out debris and rebuilding normal tissue.

The same is true in the brain. When membranes of brain cells are damaged by free radicals, proteins in the membranes trigger inflammation.

Free radicals latch onto this protein (called *arachidonic acid*) and inflammation arises. As a result, the cells are twice injured, first, directly by the free radical assault, and then indirectly by the inflammation occasioned by the rescue mission of the immune cells.

Free radicals do not exist unchecked in our systems. In the healthy body, they are neutralized and detoxified by antioxidants, almost as quickly as they are produced.

We said earlier that Alzheimer's is not caused by age, but age does play a part in leaving us susceptible to it. How great a part it plays and how vulnerable we become depends on us.

As we age, there is natural wear and tear on the brain. There is also a small amount of dehydration—our brains become slightly smaller with each decade we live—and neurons lose dendritic branches and become more simplified. The density of the synapses decreases, slowing thought. Signal transmission from one neuron to another slows as the protective covering thins.

However, nature created redundant systems of protection, and the near-infinite number of neurons, dendrites, and synapses in our brains compensates for the effect of aging on individual nerve cells. The result of fewer synapses and dendritic branches is a slowing down, not a loss, of communication between neurons in the frontal, parietal, and temporal lobes of the brain. The result is familiar to us all—the slowing down, the slackening, of thought-processes, even with all mental function intact, experienced by accelerated, unhealthy aging far beyond actual years.

Dehydration and loss of synapses only begins to occur during approximately the last third of our lives. For the first two thirds, and even during the remaining third, there are things we can do to fortify and protect our brains against Alzheimer's.

The more synapses we carry into advanced age, the more we have left as aging takes its toll. Learning, reading, exercising, and reasoning through challenging tasks all naturally increase the number of synapses in our brains. These are activities all of us can carry out, young or old. *Use it or lose it* as the saying goes, and the best way to build up any body part, including the brain and the mind, is by constant use and exercise. A bit farther on I will address preventive measures in greater detail, in addition to pointing out techniques for reducing the number of free radicals in our brains.

The first step, then, in combating Alzheimer's lies in recognizing and accepting the fact that this sickness is not the inevitable product of aging. All of us have physical and emotional challenges or problems of one variety or another, but it is necessary to realize that every problem has a solution. In fact, the solution is usually inherently found in the problem. The greatest deterrent to solving problems is fear, generally fear of unknown consequences. By gaining knowledge we may overcome that fear and develop an insight that enables us to see rational and workable solutions and to incorporate them in our daily lives.

Ralph Waldo Emerson said, "The wise man in the storm prays to God not for safety from danger, but for deliverance from fear. It is the storm within that endangers him, not the storm without."

When a person says, "I am too old," or "It cannot be done," this only means that the person is afraid to face the problem or afraid of the effort involved in taking the needed action. Remember that all problems have solutions.

Seniority can and should be the best part of life. All should be at their best, not worst, in this last phase of the cycle. Most humans do not even reach that phase or, if they do, spend it in decrepitude, bedridden, wheelchair-bound, tearful, alone, and in pain.

It was not meant to be so.

Chapter Two

Detection: The Sooner the Better

"... if the individuals have a good understanding of the disease process, the underlying causes, and the effective remedies to remove the cause, then they become active participants in their own healing process. If the underlying causes can be removed, the symptoms will follow."

—Cathy Picoulin, B.S.N., N.D., Ph.D.
Author of *Fight Alzheimer's Naturally*

Alzheimer's disease can be slowed and it can be reversed. I have seen it happen and have helped it to happen. Early detection is a huge key to successful treatment, according to Dr. Picoulin. In her naturopathic practice, Dr. Picoulin treats patients from around the world while also lecturing and writing extensively about Alzheimer's. She specializes in treating environmental toxins, parasite infestations, heavy metal overload, infections, residues, miasma, and other degenerative processes that lead to Alzheimer's.

Her knowledge has personal roots as well as scientific ones. Her own father was diagnosed with Alzheimer's, and Picoulin worked with him to reverse it.

"What if you were to find out that at least forty to fifty percent of individuals that have been diagnosed with Alzheimer's actually had a reversible condition?" Picoulin asks in her book, *Fight Alzheimer's Naturally.* "This means that your loved ones could recover most, if not all, of their cognitive abilities."

Picoulin began working with her father after he was diagnosed with Alzheimer's disease, and eight years later, his neurologist declared him free of any neurological deficits or disorders (Picoulin 2002).

"When I started this journey with my father many years ago, I was going against all odds," says Picoulin. "Alzheimer's disease was considered to be non-reversible. Brain damage was believed to be permanent. I was not willing to accept this belief. I wanted my father back."

"Today," she says of her father, "he and his wife, my mother, who worked hard making nutritional changes, have moved into the house they originally purchased to retire into. He starts up early in the morning, repairing the areas of the house that had become run down during his illness. Appliances that haven't worked in years, he is again repairing.

"His memory is sharper than my mother's, remembering every favorite actor on television," she adds. "Conversations with him reflect more insight and depth than there had been in years. His driving privileges have been returned to him, allowing him to return to his favorite golf game."

Dr. Picoulin uses an approach that employs diet and homeopathic remedies in her treatment. She explains that the main difference between conventional methods and alternative methods is that conventional methods address mostly symptoms of disease, while alternative methods work to remove the cause.

While conventional methods can be efficacious for symptom relief, until the cause of a disease is removed, the patient cannot recover. Logically, we can see that the fewer inroads a disease has been able to make, the easier it will be to remove the cause. So, early detection is a key factor in a comprehensive approach.

Warning Signs: The Earliest Detection Tool

If evening falls, and you or your loved one can't remember what room you were in when you removed your bedroom slippers that morning, should you worry that the memory lapse is caused by Alzheimer's? Perhaps. Memory lapses are one of the earliest signs of Alzheimer's, but they can also be a sign of many other dementias or age-associated memory impairments (AAMI). They can also be a sign that it has been a busy, busy day. Only professional testing can determine if Alzheimer's is the cause of the forgetfulness.

The Alzheimer's Association notes that early care and support are critical. It further notes that methods for detecting Alzheimer's have advanced in the past twenty years, to the point that professionals can make a diagnosis with more than ninety percent accuracy. This sounds a note of hope for those who may suspect that something is wrong.

The Alzheimer's Association has developed a list of warning signs that should prompt individuals or their families to seek further diagnosis:

1. **Memory Loss.**

    One of the earliest signs of dementia is forgetting recently learned information. While it's normal to forget appointments, names, or telephone numbers, those with dementia will forget such things more often and not remember them later.

2. **Difficulty Performing Familiar Tasks.**

   People with dementia often find it hard to complete everyday tasks that are so familiar we usually do not think about how to do them. A person with Alzheimer's may not know the steps for preparing a meal, using a household appliance, or participating in a lifelong hobby.

3. **Problems With Language.**

   Everyone has trouble finding the right word sometimes, but a man with Alzheimer's often forgets simple everyday words, or will substitute unusual words, making his speech or writing hard to decipher. If a woman with Alzheimer's is unable to find her toothbrush, for example, she may ask for "that thing for my mouth."

4. **Disorientation to Time and Place.**

   It's normal to forget the day of the week or where you're going, but people with Alzheimer's disease can become lost on their own street. They may forget where they are and how they got there, and may not know how to get back home.

5. **Poor or Decreased Judgment.**

   No one has perfect judgment all the time. But those with Alzheimer's may dress without regard to the weather, wearing several shirts on a warm day or very little clothing in cold temperatures. Those suffering from dementia often show poor judgment about money, giving away large sums to telemarketers or paying for home repairs or products they don't need.

6. **Problems With Abstract Thinking.**

   Balancing a checkbook is a task that can be challenging for some, but a person with Alzheimer's may forget what the numbers represent and what needs to be done with them.

7. **Misplacing Things.**

   Anyone can temporarily misplace a wallet or key. A person with Alzheimer's disease may put things in unusual places, like an iron in the freezer or a wristwatch in the sugar bowl.

8. **Changes in Mood or Behavior.**

   Everyone can become sad or moody from time to time. Someone with Alzheimer's disease can show rapid mood swings—from calm to tears to anger—for no apparent reason.

9. **Changes in Personality.**

   Personalities ordinarily change somewhat with age, but a person with Alzheimer's can metamorphose into an unknown stranger, becoming confused, suspicious, fearful, hostile, as well as childishly dependent on a family member.

10. **Loss of Initiative.**

    It's normal to tire of housework, business activities, or social obligations at times. The person with Alzheimer's disease may become very passive, sitting in front of the television for hours, sleeping more than usual, or not wanting to participate in usual activities.

Fingerprints and Other Early Markers

As a degenerative disease, Alzheimer's takes its toll gradually, and indications that abnormalities have been created surface long before memory problems occur.

Awareness of these earliest warning signs can lead an individual or his or her family to seek that very critical early professional evaluation.

Fingerprints

Research has determined that fingerprint patterns are accurate as an early marker for Alzheimer's. Patterns in fingerprints include loops, whorls, and arches, and while it is normal for them to be present, they take abnormal shapes and placement when Alzheimer's and other dementia are present.

Loops are classified as radial (pointing toward the thumb) or ulnar (pointing away from the thumb). There are also loops that point straight at the end of the finger or thumb. Straight loops are found in the non-Alzheimer's individual, as are radial loops on the index and large fingers (Weinrob, 1985).

On the hand of an individual with Alzheimer's, radial loops are found on the ring and little fingers. This person is also more likely to have ulnar loops than a healthy individual.

As I previously noted, there is no "Alzheimer's germ" whose presence could be detected with one test, so diagnosing Alzheimer's is a process of eliminating other possibilities. Therefore it is important to consider two links to other diseases when observing fingerprints as early testing for Alzheimer's:

- Whorls and arches decrease in Alzheimer's. The situation is reversed in other dementias, with an increase in these patterns.

- The same fingerprint patterns found in Alzheimer's are found in Down's Syndrome.

In the first instance, an increase in whorls and arches indicates that Alzheimer's can be excluded as part of the process-of-elimination form of diagnosis.

In the second instance, the similarity of patterns in Alzheimer's disease and Down's Syndrome probably stems from the fact that the abnormal genes for both conditions are found on the same chromosome, #19. The Down's-Alzheimer's link indicates a need for genetic testing, regardless of what other possibilities are explored, when these fingerprint patterns are present.

Sense of Smell

The individual with Alzheimer's can experience a loss of the sense of smell as early as two years before any problems with cognition become apparent. Loss of this sense can indicate that nerve cells in the olfactory lobe, the segment of the brain that controls the sense of smell, have been disrupted, damaged, or destroyed.

Testing in the home is easy. Use a variety of objects that possess distinctive odors to determine if any of this sense remains in the individual. Remember that this is a preliminary indicator and at this point, the process of elimination would have to exclude sinus trouble and other such conditions for this problem to be a true indicator of the presence of Alzheimer's.

Vision

The person with Alzheimer's may be able to see clearly but, quite early on, may not be able to interpret sights in a way that allows him to comprehend and remember. Vision problems can only be definitively identified by professionals, but a home test can show whether additional testing is necessary.

The "clock test" is a simple way to assess visual/spatial difficulties. The individual is asked to look at a clock and observe the position of the hands. Then, he or she is asked to draw the clock without seeing it.

Those with Alzheimer's will quite often draw all numbers on one side or place the clock hands in the wrong position.

Hearing

As with vision, only a professional can accurately detect physical reasons for hearing loss. However, the loss is more prevalent in Alzheimer's than in any other disease, so once possible physical causes are eliminated, it is a good marker.

Observation at home, rather than testing, is the best way to determine if hearing impairment has occurred. If the individual sets the television volume louder than is comfortable for everyone else, gets a blank look on his or her face and doesn't respond when spoken to directly, or constantly misunderstands what is being said, hearing loss is probably the case.

Depression

Like the loss of the sense of smell, depression can surface as much as two years before Alzheimer's-related memory problems appear. Sluggish behavior and morose mood are classic twin symptoms of depression. Alzheimer's should be suspected if they appear without the occurrence of a triggering event, such as the loss of a loved one, sudden financial worries, or chronic pain or illness.

Some symptoms of depression that can be observed at home are loss of interest in meals and social situations, unrelieved tiredness, crying spells, and inactivity.

Professional Testing

No test has yet been found to be one hundred percent accurate, and that is why a battery of tests is recommended in order to obtain an accurate diagnosis. It would be a daunting task, and probably ineffectual, for an individual or family to organize diagnosis by contacting various specialists and seeking myriad tests.

Therefore, once home testing and observation indicate a need for further diagnosis, the best place to start is with the family physician. The family physician can perform a thorough examination to discover or rule out physical causes for the early symptoms.

Equally important is the patient history, and the physician also learns a great deal about the memory problems by talking with the individual and his or her family. He or she may also consult a psychiatrist, psychologist or neurologist.

Neuropsychological Testing

Neuropsychological tests are a noninvasive way to appraise different areas of the brain. The individual usually takes a written test and may be asked to organize a set of sequential symbols. This tests the functioning of the frontal lobes. He or she may also be asked to take the clock test, which tests the functionality of the parietal lobes, and he or she may be tested on his or her ability to comprehend language, vocabulary, and to grasp new concepts. The latter tests the brain's temporal lobes.

Many institutions utilize neuropsychological tests whose results can only be evaluated by memory experts. These tests are complicated by the fact that they use intellectual responses to measure the physical condition of the brain, not taking into account that intellect is subject to individual experience.

For example, if someone was injured, a physician would determine the extent of the injury, to, say, the leg muscle, and a single physical standard would obtain. A limp or an inability to stand would readily indicate that the functioning of the leg muscle differed from an average, normal leg muscle.

In the case of the brain, a person's unique life experience and education color his or her intellectual responses. Therefore, the tester must work with each individual and decide what might be reasonably expected in his or her responses. Only then can a determination be made as to what constitutes a reasonable deviation from any standards or norms.

Testing for Cerebrospinal Fluid Proteins

The cerebrospinal fluid bathes the inside of the brain and the spinal cord, and its contents reflect metabolic activity in the brain. An increase or decrease in the amounts of identifiable proteins in this fluid may indicate abnormalities, such as Alzheimer's or other dementia.

Discovery of these proteins has been fairly recent. Some are already being utilized as markers in diagnostic testing, while others are still being investigated. This protein-use is novel, and represents a breakthrough in Alzheimer's diagnosis.

APP

The test for amyloid precursor protein (APP) is an instrument of exclusion. The APP, a fragment of normal amyloid protein found in the brain, becomes toxic when Alzheimer's is present, clumping and thickening in the brain. This produces a lower level of protein in the cerebrospinal fluid, which can be measured precisely via a spinal tap.

AD 7 C

The AD 7 C tests for the neural thread protein. Researchers believe the protein evolves from nerve cells in the brain and is involved in their repair and regeneration. High levels of neural thread protein are detected early in Alzheimer's, and levels climb as the disease progresses. The AD 7 C is considered ninety percent effective in diagnosing Alzheimer's and approaches autopsy in isolating the disease. This test does not require a spinal tap. It is performed on a urine sample, and results are available after forty-eight hours.

Tau Protein

A spinal tap is also required to test for tau protein, which forms as the result of degradation of nerve cells. When Alzheimer's causes abnormally high tau protein levels, they can be detected quite early on in the disease's progress. The presence of elevated tau protein is considered a strong indication that Alzheimer's may be present, though because of overlap with other dementias, it is considered a leading indicator but is not necessarily definitive.

Synaptotagmin

Researchers at Sweden's University of Göteborg have recently discovered that there is a reduction in synaptotagmin in cerebrospinal fluid and brain tissue in early-onset Alzheimer's disease. The findings are from preliminary studies, and so it is too soon to qualify as a marker or diagnostic test, but does offer promise.

AMY 117

Another potential diagnostic marker or tool, this newly discovered protein exists only in Alzheimer's patients, and is found in copious amounts within plaque-induced lesions in the brain.

AST

Aspartate aminotransferase (AST) is present only in Alzheimer's, and not in other dementias. It is produced by impaired glucose metabolism.

Imaging

Imaging is used both to determine the presence of Alzheimer's and to exclude the presence of other dementias that mask or imitate Alzheimer's. There are also many therapeutic uses for imaging. The PET scan is used in diagnosing Alzheimer's, while the CAT scan is more efficient in determining the presence of non-Alzheimer's conditions. The MRI and SPECT scans have been used successfully to diagnose Alzheimer's and exclude other dementia.

PET Scan

Positive emission tomography (PET) is the most accurate imaging technique available today. Experts speculate that 3-D PET scans will one day be able to detect obscure changes in brain metabolism, and thus predict Alzheimer's twenty years prior to its onset.

The PET scan's positron rays provide increased capabilities over X ray, magnetism, or protons. It measures blood flow, glucose utilization, oxygen consumption, and metabolism in the brain.

As is true with much of new technology, the PET scan is both expensive and severely limited in availability, but, as is true with all new technologies, its cost can be expected to drop and its availability to increase in the course of time.

SPECT Scan

Single photon emission computed tomography (SPECT) should be mentioned here because it is an imaging technique, but its precision is not as accurate as other methods in diagnosing Alzheimer's. There is a newer, three-dimensional SPECT scan that is more accurate, and it is best used for a perfusion test of the temporoparietal area of the brain.

A perfusion test measures how rapidly and effectively blood passes through the tissue under examination. By clearly showing the actual flow of blood into tissues, the SPECT finds defects and structural changes in this area of the brain.

CAT Scan

Computed axial tomography (CAT) is more accurate in imaging circulatory disease and strokes than it is for diagnosing Alzheimer's, and so it is a tool for exclusion.

MRI

Magnetic resonance imaging (MRI) works best in early detection of atrophy of the hippocampal and temporal lobes. Because Alzheimer's symptoms do not become apparent until much damage has been done, the ability to measure these parts of the brain by volume using MRI is an invaluable tool in early diagnosis. The temporal lobes show up very well in MRI also.

EEG

Brain waves slow in other diseases besides Alzheimer's, so while electroencephalogram (EEG) tests are helpful in indicating that a problem exists, they cannot be used to specifically detect the presence of Alzheimer's.

BEAM

As with the EEG, brain electrical activity mapping (BEAM) can also uncover a problem, in this case by measuring brain wave velocity. However, it cannot differentiate Alzheimer's from other causes, such as anxiety, depression, alcohol and cocaine abuse, and Parkinson's disease.

Blood Testing

Blood testing is used for the process of elimination, by detecting other conditions that can mask or mimic Alzheimer's. Red and white blood cell counts are measured, in addition to the levels of hormones, B12, folate, and thyroid. Blood testing is needed to rule out the presence of HIV, drugs, and heavy metals, among others.

No test, however sophisticated, is totally accurate, and autopsy is the only definite method of determining if Alzheimer's is present. In the absence of absolute certainty, these tests, taken together, provide the professional with enough information to indicate that treatment for Alzheimer's should begin. To further clarify, if an individual is suspected to have Alzheimer's but the diagnosis is not 100% certain, a question naturally arises: should treatment begin? The answer is a resounding yes, because the proper treatment for Alzheimer's is to implement a natural, healthy lifestyle, eliminating the cause of disease. This will promote health and aid recovery from *any* degenerative illness.

Chapter Three

Immunity and Alzheimer's

"Immunity IS Prevention"
—Dr. A. I. Anbar, 1954

It is easy to see how adding abundant, proper nutrients to our diets will aid in strengthening the body's immunity. If we do this, we will have won half the battle for cellular health. The other half of the battle, though it may not sound difficult, is much tougher: avoiding substances detrimental to cell health.

Some of the culprits can be found in the very foods we seek for healthful nutrients. Along with our beneficial foods, fruits, vegetables, legumes and nuts, we are liable to also take in a heavy dose of pesticides, herbicides, antibiotics, fertilizers, artificial colorings and flavor and appearance enhancers. To their credit, consumers have become increasingly aware of the presence of these toxic hitchhikers in their food supply, and the demand for organically-grown produce has boosted sales in this market substantially in recent years. In response, mainstream food chains have

31

begun to devote more and more shelf space to a wider variety of organically grown foods.

Not coincidentally, consumer action groups have successfully demanded nutritional changes in food served to school children, many of whom are obese and hyperactive (the result of too much sugar and fat) and are working to obtain healthier, less fattening fare for school lunches. Restaurants, too, have become part of their focus. Here they have been more successful in raising public awareness of ingredients used in preparing meals than in actually forcing changes in quality and preparation. Still, the situation is somewhat better than in the recent past.

While these developments in the market signal a turn, or return, to healthy eating habits for part of the population, Americans as a whole are not headed in this direction. Unlike the Hunza philosophy, there is no unified American attitude that embraces eating foods in their natural state.

In fact, the market for junk food and other detrimental fare has far outdistanced sales of the organic. With all the nutritional and health information available to Americans, this phenomenon of a national taste for toxicity is as curious as it is lethal. It would take another book to explain it, but suffice it to say for our purposes that the attraction is fueled by social structure, negative financial interests, and the food's intrinsic nature.

Fat and Salt: The Evil Twins

Fat and salt are appetite-whetters that keep us coming back for more. Fat partners with salt for the total no-no taste experience. Although salt is a necessary nutrient, it is so pervasive in our diets, so pumped and loaded into every food, particularly the prepackaged types, that we need to become very discerning ingredient-readers if we hope to keep our intake within a healthy range.

Fat presents a dual threat. It swells the number of free

radicals in our bodies, while also inducing a chemical change that actually makes us crave even more fat, resulting in a never-ending cycle of destructive overeating.

Metabolism of large quantities of fats causes increased oxidation and free radicals and subsequent damage to mitochondria. Damaged mitochondria then cannot produce adenosine triphosphate (ATP), which is energy-essential for electron transfer in neurons. Without nerve impulses, our cells die.

Fats contribute to free radical production at different rates, depending upon whether they are polyunsaturated, monosaturated, or polysaturated. These names reflect whether none, one, or all sites on the fat molecule are bound.

All animal fats contribute to oxidation and should be avoided as much as possible, and saturated fats should be omitted altogether from the diet. (One quick way to identify and therefore avoid these is to remember that fats which are solid at room temperature are always saturated.) In fact, one of the messages that Alzheimer's disease holds for us is that the vegetarian diet, or the Hunza-style vegetable-dominated diet, is a key to health.

Essential Fatty Acids

Omega-3 and omega-6 fatty acids should be kept in the diet, however. We need these for survival. In fact, they are known as essential fatty acids (EFAs). As we have seen with other nutrients, omega-3 and omega-6 work in relationship to each other, and the relative amounts of EFAs present in our bodies have an impact on our cells. When the amount of omega-6 fatty acid significantly outweighs the amount of omega-3, the body reduces production of needed DHA (a long-chain omega-3 produced from short-chain dietary omega-3).

The typically meat-loaded American diet promotes this imbalance, because omega-6 fatty acids are found in animal

products. Sufficient daily omega-3 intake can be assured by
making sure the diet includes some of the following:

Flaxseed	1 tablespoon
Flax oil	1 tablespoon
English Walnuts	12 walnut halves
Soybeans (green, frozen, or raw)	1-1/2 cup
Tofu	1-1/2 cup

Avoiding eating fats is not as easy as it sounds. Eating fats is
a habit with most of us and, like all habits, it is difficult to break.
We encounter many factors that trigger our hunger for fat. These
may be events, such as lunch with coworkers and family or holi-
day dinners, or emotions brought on by positive or negative
experiences that send us to the "comfort" food.

Brain chemistry also plays a part in our including fat in our
diet. Desire for food is influenced by neurotransmitters, and
when these neurotransmitters, such as serotonin, are
depressed, cravings result.

Paradoxically, sensitivity or allergy to fat also can cause us
to crave fat, in the same psychological way that alcohol and
cigarettes can make us want them.

For example, the first-time drinker is only too aware of
alcohol as a component of the drink: one first-timer reported
that she thought that paint thinner might taste a whole lot like
her first cocktail. Yet, the feeling of euphoria produced by consuming alcohol often overcomes the first aversion to the taste
and stimulates an interest in drinking.

So it is with food sensitivity to fat. When those who are sensitive to fat consume it, endorphins are released, giving us a
"feel-good" sensation, which we then begin to crave. This "feel-
good" sensation can become the basis of addiction.

Now, picture our addicted selves at large in the world,

bombarded by advertising for fat-laden food, which is constantly within easy reach at fast-food and coffee/baked goods counters, at eat-in restaurants, for take-out and delivery, in supermarkets, on the office "share" table, and in the homes of our friends and ourselves. Is it any wonder that the fat habit is difficult to break?

Stress and Immunity

Scientists have long known that stress affects the immune system as the body responds to disruptive outside influences that may be psychological, physical, or a combination of both. They have also found that, depending on the situation, stress can either boost our immune system or suppress it.

A good example of this can be seen in the link between the high-stress response life lived by the "Type A"(and newly classified "Type D" person, *Newsweek*, October 2005) and the breakdown of that person's immune system, resulting in coronary heart disease. This link contains strong implications for those seeking ways to avoid or reverse Alzheimer's.

None of us can avoid stress; indeed, some of it is essential to survival. For example, it is our reaction to immediate stress that propels us into the street when our toddler wanders off the sidewalk. Known as "fight or flight," this reaction gets us moving when only quick and immediate action can rescue him from the path of an oncoming car.

Two Types of Immune Responses

There are two types of immune responses, which scientists have termed natural and specific. The responses vary in the method they use to fight off attackers and the amount of time they require to do so.

Natural immunity allows a quick response to invasion. The cells it produces provide protection of a general nature. These cells can ward off a wide range of pathogens, and their work is characterized by fever and inflammation. Researchers have found that the fight or flight immune response prepares to defend the body because the body has been breached; it does not matter if the injury has been caused by accident or by intent.

Specific immunity requires more time to take effect, but it is able to produce protection cells that are tailored to the specific invader. Several days are required for specific immunity to recognize an invader and respond with specialized cells. This includes the lymphocytes, which are T-cells and B-cells. Specific immunity responds appropriately to cellular stressors, such as viruses, which penetrate cells, and humoral stressors, such as bacteria and parasites, which remain outside the cells.

Many Types of Stress

It is the nature of the stress encountered rather than the type of immune response, which determines whether the immune system will function properly or begin to break down. When the stress is prolonged and assumes the nature of a siege, the immune system undergoes radical changes, and can eventually cease to function altogether. This phenomenon is linked to an individual's perception of whether or not the stress will end.

When stress is short-term, the fight or flight response handles the threat, and the episode is concluded. This is the response we see when a child's skinned knee or an athlete's lacerated body heals and the damage disappears.

In an interesting study appearing in the July 2005 issue of the *Psychological Bulletin*, published by the American Psychological Association, researchers Suzanne Segerstrom, Ph.D., and Gregory Miller, Ph.D., divided stressors into types defined by their nature and duration.

Two types of short-term stress identified by the researchers are those they call acute time-limited stressors, which include such things as public speaking, and brief naturalistic stressors, which include challenges like academic tests. As stressful as most people might find such situations, they can expect these events to conclude in a relatively short time. Underscoring this latter idea in *The Biology of Belief,* a groundbreaking new book demonstrating how our bodies can be transformed as we re-program our thinking, Bruce Lipton, a former medical school professor, tells of the terror struck into medical students by his distributing pop quizzes, with no advance warning. So stressful did the students consider the situation that their scores were far lower than when they had prior warning of a test, even though the questions and material were nearly identical. People who do not "test well" actually mean that their minds are preoccupied with their fear above all else. They are too busy projecting negative results and repercussions to process and transmit the information they already possess.

Segerstrom and Miller identify long-term stressors as chronic or distant. Chronic stressors affect a person's total life, either in terms of how they identify themselves or how they are able to conduct themselves in social interactions. There is also no end in sight for these situations. Examples of people who are chronically stressed are those whose injuries have produced habitual pain, or persons living in a war zone.

Unlike chronic stressors, the immediate causes of distant stressors have been removed, but their influence has survived and continues to interfere with a person's daily life. As an example, someone affected by distant stress might be a former prisoner of war, or someone who had suffered abuse during childhood.

Segerstrom and Miller also found that bridging the long-term and short-term stressors are stressful event sequences, major events such as death of a loved one or hurricane or some other natural disaster devastating a community. These events are more significant and disruptive than the typical short-term stressors, but they can be expected to come to a conclusion.

The researchers have noted that the immune system seems to be affected somewhat by stressful event sequences, but the link between chronic stressors and suppression of the immune system is evident. When chronic stress is present, all immune functions are affected, and the longer it continues, the more the system becomes suppressed.

Taking the Stress out of Stress

Stories abound about tough-guy radio host G. Gordon Liddy, and how he got that way. Most prevalent is the tale of how he overcame a fear of rats: he caught one, cooked it, and ate it. The trick, he advises, is not to mind it.

It would follow, then, that the way to avoid being made ill by stress is ... not to be bothered by stress. Contradictory as it sounds, this is exactly the way to combat this killer. It is our *response* to stressors that triggers our physical reactions, not the events themselves.

The Nun Study

Preliminary findings from the study of a religious community in relation to Alzheimer's indicate that there may be a link between attitude and immunity strength. Dubbed the Nun Study, this ongoing inquiry found that participants who displayed a positive outlook on life tended to outlive those who were less optimistic.

Nearly twenty years ago David Snowdon, a neurologist, conducted a study of 700 members of the School Sisters of Notre Dame. The sisters, aged 75 to 102 years when the study began, agreed to be tested for cognitive function each year, to have annual physical examinations, and to donate their brains for study at their deaths.

Researchers had access to autobiographies written by 180 of the sisters at the time they took their vows; their ages ranged from 18 to the mid-30s when they wrote them. Although the majority of that group lived to an advanced age, the nuns who revealed a positive outlook as young women lived to an average of 94, about eight years longer than their less positive sisters.

There are some limitations to the study. The group is homogenous, with lives that are identical in major aspects such as socialization, career, and type and availability of health care. For this reason researchers are cautious about applying the findings to the public in general. However, for these same reasons, findings within the group are clearer because individual experience carries so little weight as a variable. Researchers have yet to regard results of the Nun Study as conclusive, and so it is ongoing, already having revealed another hidden message from Alzheimer's.

The Mind Matters

How did the long-living nuns arrive at their emotionally serene status? Were their lives somehow freer of stress than those experienced by the rest of us, or had they discovered effective ways to cope with stress, even at their young ages? Observers hope the Nun Study may be able to answer these questions as research continues. We can hope that the conclusions will translate into helpful news for the rest of the population.

Even now, a variety of methods are at our disposal that will help us avoid putting our immune system on full combat alert when the unavoidable stresses of life arise. Physical exercise, meditation, and other psychophysiological techniques all can help relieve stress. Counseling and therapy also may be indicated for dealing with acute and long-term stressors.

Taking Charge of Our Stress

The scene is the emergency room of a city hospital on a typical Saturday night. Wailing in the waiting room is a toddler with a marble up his nose. His young, inexperienced mother is standing at the sign-in desk, approaching the wailing point herself and begging for attention for her baby. Already signed in, a Little Leaguer cradles his injured arm with his good one, and a woman six months pregnant groans as premature contractions wrack her body. Then, the bay doors bang open as paramedics wheel in the first of four victims of an automobile accident.

If the medical personnel on duty reacted to the disturbance the way many of our bodies react to stress, none of the patients would have a chance. Even though we are responsible for this one life, ours, stressors can set off so much demand for attention from our body and mind that we do not know what to deal with first and confusion and, often, panic result.

Triage: A Planned Response to Stressors

The way an emergency room deals with the unpredictable and urgent nature of its business shows us a way to deal with our own stress. First, emergency personnel use a method called triage, from the French for "to sift out." Cases are prioritized according to their seriousness, with the most urgent cases attended to first. Then, they are assigned to the appropriate area, such as a regular treatment room or the operating room. Then, the appropriate equipment and personnel are assembled, anyone from a lowly intern with a stethoscope to a surgeon with all the sophisticated equipment he or she will require.

Personnel are able to step in confidently and do what needs to be done because they know that they have the tools and training to do so and that they have a plan for using them. So it should be with us in times of stress.

As the Segerstrom-Miller study indicates, situations that leave us feeling hopeless and powerless produce the stress that is most harmful to our immune system. When faced with the unexpected or stressful situation, we can conduct our own triage that allows us to take charge, if only of our responses to it.

That is a crucial point to remember. *When we say we are working to control stress in our lives, we are working on the only aspect of it that is truly within our control: our response to it.*

It has been one of those weeks. Last-minute changes from a client have had you at work early and late every day. Each day, you have only been home long enough to eat something and fall into bed, dressing quickly and leaving for work again a few short hours later. The hard work paid off, however. The project was finished on time this morning, even though it took working on Saturday. The client is very pleased, and there is talk of bonuses.

Now, it's Saturday afternoon. All those clothes you discarded this week are in the hamper, and you're going to have to do some laundry before you head back in on Monday. There isn't much of anything to eat in the house, either, so a trip to the grocery store is on your to-do list for today. Later. For the first time since last weekend, there is nothing pressing that demands your immediate attention. The sun is shining, and you're just going to sit here and bask in it and the memory of a job well done. You feel the tensions of the week easing out of your neck and shoulder muscles, and a wonderful feeling of well-being envelopes you.

The doorbell rings. Some of your friends from work, still

excited from this week's triumph, are at your door. They have organized an impromptu picnic to celebrate the successful project, and they are laden with coolers containing food and drinks. Apartment dwellers, they reasoned that since you are the only one in the group who lives in a house with a backyard, you wouldn't mind hosting the celebration.

Stressors galore have suddenly invaded your peaceful afternoon. If these people begin a party now, they'll still be here long after nightfall. You'll have to drag out the extra folding chairs and little yard tables you usually use for a party in the yard. They didn't remember to bring paper plates or plastic silverware. You think you have some picnic supplies from last summer stashed in the back of a cabinet somewhere. You hope they brought enough food, because you're desperately running your mind over what you have in the house, and there is nothing that can make a contribution to this party.

Now, you're going to have to do your laundry and shopping tomorrow. You need to clean house and pay bills, too. Suddenly, you can see Monday looming right in front of you, and you are still as fatigued as you were Friday night. You can feel your neck and shoulders tensing up again.

As you can see, there is nothing you can do about the cause of stress. You had no control over these stressors, in the form of your exuberant coworkers, showing up on your doorstep. All you can do is control how you respond to this situation.

Remember the triage approach. The guiding principle is that you have the resources necessary to deal with stressful situations. Knowing this allows you to calmly assess the event and make decisions.

Remove the Stressor

Almost always, your first option is not to participate in stress-making activity. It is perfectly reasonable, and your right, to decline to host this impromptu event. You have the right to claim fatigue, prior commitments, or whatever applies, as you send the party elsewhere, all the while expressing regret that you'll miss out on the fun, of course. They can have their picnic in a park, perhaps, but in any case, it is not your responsibility. If these people want to have a party, you can be assured that they will have one.

This option if often overlooked or discounted when, as in some serious situations, it should be the first choice. For example, you may be searching for ways to cope with stress because you know it is causing your work to deteriorate and your friendships and family ties to wither. If the cause of this stress is an abusive relationship in which you find yourself, then by all means, remove yourself from the abusive environment, or remove the abuser from your environment. You can see that if you're not under any obligation to host a party, you certainly do not have to accept abuse.

Calmly Assess the Situation

So, what if you don't choose to simply remove the source of stress? What if there is a reason for you to be in a situation with a potential for causing you stress? For example, these are your friends, who simply want to share their happiness with you and credit you with helping to bring it about. You would like to celebrate with them, if you weren't worried about taking care of everything else.

First step of triage is to prioritize the seriousness of the situation. How serious is an unplanned party? Not dangerous or life threatening. Haste and fear or worry are not required to deal with it, so you can relax.

Assign to the Proper Area

In many cases, as in this one, once you begin to assess a situation, you will see that segments of it are already well in hand, and you don't have to deal with them. In this instance, your friends have only asked to use your backyard. You don't have to worry that your house isn't ready for company. Emotionally, this is the same as not having to play the beleaguered admissions desk clerk at that emergency room. Your friends have already decided that a simple treatment room will do.

Assemble Personnel and Equipment

Other people are one of our greatest resources for preventing stress, and asking for help is something many of us find most difficult to do. Is it really necessary for you to run around, setting up picnic furniture, lighting the grill, and carrying out eating utensils? Of course not. Your friends organized a group, gathered up their contributions to the party, and got themselves to your house. They are ready and eager to put this thing together. Put them to work.

Okay, that takes care of the possible stress of hosting this party. What of your other concerns? By keeping your sense of humor and thinking creatively, you may find a solution for them, also.

You can't really ask your friends to clean your house before they have a party, and you wouldn't want them involved in your bill paying, but the party and your concerns do have a common denominator in the grocery store. Task someone with setting out drinks and chips and other snacks the group might have brought. Ask someone else to get the grill ready and "guest host" for you for a little while. Grab a friend who works well with you and your grocery list and head for the store. Once there, cut the list in half and send your friend after half the items while you cover the others, to meet at the checkout so you can pay for them. While you're getting your groceries, grab some salad in a bag and a variety of dressings, or frozen snacks you can quickly prepare in the oven when you get home. Now, you have your contribution to the party, and your shopping is completed. That makes the remaining tasks seem manageable for the next day—and if your friend's interpretation of your list yields brands or items different from what you usually purchase, you may discover something new that you really enjoy.

Of course, as with opting out of a stressful situation, dealing with it has implications for more serious events, such as caring for a parent or spouse with Alzheimer's, as well as for social occasions that may be merely annoying.

Then, assessing the situation deals with determining how severe the effects of Alzheimer's have become, and that information is needed to assign to the proper area (home or health care center), and assemble appropriate personnel (ask for emotional help as well as help with physical tasks from friends and family). Equipment needed to deal with serious situations may also include our religious or spiritual resources.

To recap, our triage for dealing with stress:

- Expect to encounter stressors. That's life. We can't avoid them.

- Stay calm. Remember that you have resources and a plan.

- Consider removing the stressor. Some situations are not our responsibility.

- Calmly assess the situation. Is the source of stress a life or death situation, or more of a social nature?

- Assign to the proper area. This can be a physical place or our mental setting of emotions.

- Assemble appropriate personnel and equipment. Ask for help. Draw on beliefs in addition to training and experience.

The Genetic Message

For a small portion of the population, the message of Alzheimer's has a genetic significance. The group affected is not large—only about twenty percent of those who contract Alzheimer's carry the predisposition to the disease—but the message is clear: if someone in your family has Alzheimer's, the chances are that you carry the vulnerability to it in your genes.

The affected genes are not the disease. They merely represent vulnerability, and it is not inevitable that the person affected contract Alzheimer's, especially if the immune system is properly supported.

Also, genetic researchers are greatly increasing the body of knowledge in this area, and they have identified genes responsible for the onset of various forms of Alzheimer's. The cause of some forms of both late and early-onset Alzheimer's can be found in genes, but the earlier the onset, the more likely genetics have played a part. Discovery of these genes has enabled scientists to develop possible gene therapies which are in the early stages of testing.

How Genes Work

To understand how genes can leave one open to contracting Alzheimer's, it is important to understand how they work under normal circumstances. Genes are comprised of DNA (deoxyribonucleic acid), and the DNA found in each gene is identical. Genes occur in pairs, half of each pair having been donated by each parent.

Genes make up chromosomes, and there are twenty-three pairs of chromosomes in each cell in the body. Each chromosome is built of thousands of genes, and there are more than 50,000 genes in each cell.

Mutation: A Damaged Inheritance

It is through the DNA that we receive our family characteristics and pass them on to future generations. Most of the time, any difference between us and other generations in our family is merely a matter of dominance or recessiveness of certain genes. It doesn't matter which generation develops the characteristic—blue eyes, for example—the genes are passed on by preceding generations.

For instance, the gene for blue eyes is recessive. That means that it is weaker than a dominant gene, such as the gene for brown eyes. So, both genes in the pair must be for blue eyes in order for the individual to have blue eyes. The genes for blue eyes came through the generations, from blue-eyed ancestors with two recessive genes for blue eyes or from brown-eyed individuals who carried one recessive gene for blue eyes and one dominant gene for brown eyes. This stronger gene makes itself known in the outward, brown-eyed appearance.

Embryos grow and develop by cells dividing and growing. Under normal circumstances, DNA copies itself exactly with each division and each new cell has the same chromosomal and genetic makeup.

In mutation, genes are altered from the familial heritage and become the first generation of a new gene, which is then passed on to succeeding generations. This occurs because there is an error when the DNA copies itself for the new cell.

Mutations and Alzheimer's

Not all mutations are harmful, but vulnerability to Alzheimer's is possible when mutations affect genes that control proteins in the body.

There are many different proteins in the body, and each is normally controlled by a pair of genes. Mutation can cause one gene of the pair to make an extra copy or allele of itself, disrupting the function of the paired genes and, in consequence, the makeup of the protein in their control. Mutation can occur in both genes of the pair. All alleles are passed on to succeeding generations.

Genetic Factors in Early-Onset Alzheimer's

Most people who develop the disease have late-onset Alzheimer's, and their symptoms do not usually develop until they are in their seventies. Individuals with early-onset Alzheimer's can develop symptoms as early as their forties or fifties.

Scientists are still intensely researching the genetic connection to Alzheimer's, and so far have identified mutated genes on three chromosomes, numbers 1, 14, and 21. Little information is available as yet, but scientists are studying chromosomes 4, 6, and 20 for possible links to Alzheimer's.

Amyloid Precursor Protein (APP)

When the mutation affects the gene that controls amyloid precursor protein, there may be an increase in production or deposits of beta amyloid, the material at the core of neuritic plaques. This mutation has been identified as the cause of a relatively small amount, only two to three percent, of early-onset Alzheimer's cases.

The amyloid precursor protein (APP) gene is found on chromosome 21. Amyloid is a normal protein found in the brain. It has a tendency to become toxic by several processes, including mutation. Toxic amyloid forms clumps on nerve cell receptors. Thus, it is labeled a precursor of the abnormal plaque formations between brain cells characteristic of Alzheimer's disease. The mutant gene controls APP's rate of the toxicity that forms plaque.

This toxicity causes a marker used to diagnose Alzheimer's:

when APP clumps in the brain, its levels in the cerebrospinal fluid correspondingly decrease in measurable amounts. Lowered APP levels in the cerebrospinal fluid correspond to decreased cognition.

H2LA-2A Gene

The H2LA-2A gene is thought to be responsible for a form of early-onset Alzheimer's by its role in inflammation. This gene is considered responsible for Alzheimer's appearance two to four years earlier in patients who carry it, compared to patients who do not possess it. Much more remains to be learned about this gene, but researchers are studying its response to anti-inflammatories.

Presenilin 1 and 2

Two other mutated genes, called the presenilins, have been identified in relation to early-onset Alzheimer's. Presenilin 1 is found on chromosome 14 and presenilin 2 is found on chromosome 1.

Seventy percent of patients suffering from early-onset Alzheimer's have been found to have the presenilin 1 gene. Individuals feel its effect between the ages of thirty and sixty-five. Scientists have found forty-two mutations on this gene.

Presenilin 2 accounts for 25 percent of those individuals contracting early-onset Alzheimer's. Scientists have found two mutations on this gene.

The presenilin alleles are thought to contribute to Alzheimer's by causing oxidative stress in the brain. Affected brain cells then give up calcium. These activities disrupt the mitochondria and consequently the electron transfer between cells. Deprived of this essential energy, nerves degenerate and die.

Antioxidants such as vitamin E are considered effective

means to counteract the effects of the presenilin alleles. There has also been some success in slowing the progression of the disease with calcium channel blockers, which are prescription medicines widely used to treat high blood pressure and angina.

Genes Affect Late-Onset Alzheimer's

While early-onset Alzheimer's is a clear sign that genetics are probably playing a part in the disease, mutations have also been associated with some forms of late-onset Alzheimer's. In the past, the early-onset forms were considered to be the only forms whose causes lay in genetics.

However, as with all science, medical knowledge evolves and more breakthroughs are made. With the latest advances and theories, vulnerability to late-onset as well as early-onset Alzheimer's is thought to have genetic causes. In fact, among the newest discoveries is a mutant gene on chromosome 12 that may be responsible for as much as fifteen percent of late-onset cases.

Cytochrome C Oxidase Gene: The Maternal Influence

When either parent contracts Alzheimer's, children can consider that they may have inherited a mutant gene that leaves them vulnerable to the disease. Children of mothers with Alzheimer's are much more likely to develop the disease than children whose fathers are affected.

This allele is caused by a mutation of the DNA of the mitochondria, which provides power to the cells. This mutation is nine times as likely to occur in the cells of the female parent, compared to the cells of the male parent. Correspondingly, children of mothers with Alzheimer's are nine times more likely to develop the disease than children of fathers with the disease.

Apolipoprotein E (APOE)

Apolipoprotein E (APOE) is found on chromosome 19 and its function is tied to transport of cholesterol. It is found in four types, whose associations with Alzheimer's are varied.

There are three forms of APOE whose effects are thought to be benign, and possibly even protective, as far as Alzheimer's is concerned:

- Apolipoprotein E1 (APOE 1). This type offers protection against coronary disease and heart attacks. At this time, there is no known association with Alzheimer's.

- Apolipoprotein E2 (APOE 2). Research continues on this allele, thought by some to be instrumental in holding off the onset of Alzheimer's, or at least not to cause early onset. Conflicting results have been produced by studies of the survival rates of those who carry the allele, and its function regarding Alzheimer's has not yet been fully discovered.

- Apolipoprotein E3 (APOE 3) appears to be neutral, having little effect on the development or protection against Alzheimer's.

Apolipoprotein E4 (APOE 4) is the harmful allele. In addition to creating vulnerability genetically, it is also linked to sporadic categories of late-onset Alzheimer's. It is thought to be responsible for about seventy percent of both familial and sporadic late-onset Alzheimer's dementia.

It is believed that more than thirty percent of all Americans have one allele of APOE 4. This creates a vulnerability, if small, toward developing the disease. It is estimated that ten percent of those carrying one extra copy of this gene will develop

Alzheimer's, compared to the ninety percent who will not contract the disease.

The chances of developing Alzheimer's increase dramatically when one more allele is present. Then there is an even chance, fifty percent, that those individuals will develop it. Fortunately for most, only about two percent of the population carry dual copies of this gene.

APOE 4's pervasiveness intensifies in the presence of other conditions. For example, if a person who has inherited the allele suffers head trauma, he or she is ten times as likely to develop Alzheimer's-related dementia. APOE 4 is thought to be less effective than E2 or E3 in repairing damage to the brain after trauma. So people with extra copies of the gene are more susceptible to memory problems after a stroke.

As with the allele for the cytochrome C oxidase gene, there seems to be an effect based on gender. The effect is still under study, but early indications are that men with Alzheimer's who have inherited APOE 4 may not survive quite as long as women under the same conditions. The difference in survival time between the two groups seems to be slight, but the ramifications warrant further study.

Individuals with herpes meningitis (inflammation of the lining of the brain caused by the herpes virus) also face more risk when they have inherited the APOE 4 allele. There is a much higher incidence of dementia when both the allele and meningitis are present.

Apolipoprotein C 1

Also located on chromosome 19, this gene has been found close to apolipoprotein E. Still under study, it is considered a source of vulnerability to Alzheimer's. Genetic vulnerability and immunity play a decisive role in developing or preventing Alzheimer's.

Chapter Four

The Role of Exercise in Prevention and Treatment

When we begin to understand the message of Alzheimer's, we realize that being healthy is a choice we can make for ourselves. Once we have chosen to be healthy, it is time to get going—literally.

For centuries, medical professionals and laypersons alike have recognized that physical exercise plays a huge part in maintaining health. It is only recently, however, that we have come to understand that exercise is *absolutely essential* to good health. The U.S. Centers for Disease Control and Prevention recently predicted that if the tendency of today's children to eat poorly and to lack exercise is not reversed, they will be the first generation to live shorter lives than their parents. This is a frightening statement. In fact, researchers in almost every medical and scientific field are coming to the conclusion that exercise saves lives. Their reports are being made public and are arriving with alarming frequency.

USC, Irvine

The Journal of Neuroscience reported recently on work by Paul Adlard and other researchers at the University of California at Irvine, using genetically engineered mice that at the age of three months developed plaques, the clumps of amyloid protein that are characteristic of Alzheimer's.

There were running wheels in the cages of half the mice. The other cages contained no such apparatus. The mice were tested in their ability to navigate a water maze. The mice which had access to the running wheels learned to navigate the maze faster than the mice which had been inactive.

In addition, at autopsy the researchers found fewer plaques and beta-amyloid peptides in the brains of the mice which had exercised. The difference between the two groups was significant in the amount of the substances characteristic of Alzheimer's that were found, even though both groups had begun to show the signs of Alzheimer's before the test began.

The study was partially funded by the National Institute on Aging, whose spokesperson, Stephen Snyder, an expert on Alzheimer's, said, "These results suggest that exercise—a simple behavioral strategy—in these mice may bring about a change in the way that amyloid precursor protein is metabolized."

Brain Institute, the University of Queensland, Australia

Perry Bartlett, a professor and researcher at the Brain Institute, reported recently that mental and physical exercise appears to promote growth of new brain cells. He reported that a chemical called prolactin supports the growth of new cells. He stated that new cell growth could help prevent dementia and other degenerative diseases.

Bartlett also noted that prolactin levels, which he found to be elevated in pregnant women, also rise during physical activity.

The Mayo Clinic

Experts on aging at the Mayo Clinic report that exercise imparts emotional and physical benefits to Alzheimer's patients as well as to other aging individuals.

"Improved strength, endurance and cardiovascular health, and help with controlling blood pressure are known benefits of exercise," Janet Vittone, a geriatrician at the clinic, reported recently. "In addition, exercise may reduce the risk of falls and fractures in older adults. Time spent exercising with someone with Alzheimer's also enhances emotional bonding."

There are many benefits that all can derive from exercise, whether they are afflicted with a degenerative disease or not. In addition, exercise can give a sense of purpose and meaning to the Alzheimer's patient, whose life has often become shrunken and limited due to the disease. In this way, exercise has a calming effect. There are also other physical benefits, of special concern to the Alzheimer's patient. Exercise improves energy, circulation, stamina, and mood; improves sleep; aids in elimination and reduces constipation; and helps the sufferer retain and even enhance motor skills. The patient may also be at reduced risk for injury in the case of a fall, since exercise sustains and helps to increase strength, flexibility, and balance.

"If the person with Alzheimer's is in the earlier stage of the disease, weight training could be added to benefit his or her strength and balance," Dr. Vittone reported. "Depending upon the progression of the disease, close observation during such exercise likely will be necessary."

Exercise Hints for Caregivers

There are certain factors that caregivers must consider before
and during an exercise regimen for those in their charge. Of
primary concern are any medical conditions that may impact
the person's ability to exercise. Consult the individual's physician before embarking on any exercise program.

Once cleared medically, remember that persons with
Alzheimer's may approach exercise with energy and enthusiasm
but may be unable to choose or organize appropriate activities.
The caregiver must be the leader in this area, arranging activities
in safe and congenial surroundings. Remember, too, that the
exercise area should be free of distractions which could cause confusion and frustration for the Alzheimer's individual. The caregiver should be present at all times during any exercise, to give support and maintain supervision.

Dr. Vittone wisely suggested that an exercise program begin
with an activity that the patient enjoyed in the past, which might
be something as simple as walking or something more strenuous,
like swimming. She also reminded caregivers to tailor goals to the
patients' abilities, keeping activities within their comfort zone
and encouraging their efforts.

The Mayo Clinic offers the following tips for keeping exercise safe, as well as fun:

To ensure safety and comfort during exercise:

- You both should dress according to the weather;
  layers of clothing work best in cool weather.

- Wear comfortable shoes.

- Keep instructions and directions simple.

- Remember to begin with mild stretching exercises
  for the upper and middle body.

- Show the person under your care how to relax by first tensing, then releasing, various muscle groups.
- Be the leader. Ask your charge to follow your example in exercising.
- Consult a doctor if the individual mentions pain, dizziness, or shortness of breath.
- Once begun, safeguard the routine:
- Exercise regularly. In bad weather, take a trip to the mall or other inside facility for a walk, or walk inside your home.
- Perform exercises in the same sequence during each period.
- Minimizing confusion is essential. Use the same route for walking each time.
- Whenever possible, conduct the exercise session at the same time each day.

Use some imagination and creativity to spark interest in exercise.

- Plug in an exercise tape or disc and help your charge to follow along.
- Teach activities that interest the individual as a springboard to exercise. This could be anything from dancing to going on a walk and bird-watching.
- Memory cues are essential. For example, when dancing is the exercise, choose music that is significant and enjoyable for the patient.
- Tailor activities and create movement sequences if full activity is no longer possible. For example, if

the person used to be an avid golfer, going a full
eighteen holes is probably now impossible, but he
or she might enjoy practicing putting in the yard;
or a former bicyclist may enjoy sharing the ride
on a tandem.

- Make it a social occasion. Exercise along with your
charge, and seek out exercise groups if he or she is
comfortable meeting with others.

Above all, be realistic. Do not expect success of Olympian
proportions. You must, however, see that your charge can sustain
his or her ability to move well enough to tend to his or her own
grooming needs. He or she may also be able to perform light
household chores. All of this will give him or her a feeling of
belonging, of usefulness and independence, and a sense of purpose in the household.

The clinic further reported that caregivers can also benefit
from the experience since it means engaging in physical activity
themselves. In a study of women who cared for a relative with
dementia, researchers found that exercising four times per week
improved the emotional and physical health of the caregivers.
Blood pressure went down, sleeping improved, and feelings of
stress and depression abated.

The American Dietetic Association

The American Dietetic Association has concluded a field trial
that measured the health benefits of modifying not only diet
but physical activity through education. Writing in their association's journal researchers reported on a randomized clinical
trial comprising 337 volunteers who ranged in age from 43 to
81. The group was drawn from the metropolitan area of
Rockford, Illinois.

Volunteers were divided into two groups, a control group

and an intervention group. The intervention group attended a forty-hour educational course in which they were taught the importance of making healthy choices regarding diet and exercise, and also were taught how to make good choices. The control group did not receive the education.

At the beginning of the study and again at six weeks, researchers assessed all the volunteers for health knowledge as well as actual practices in diet and exercise, and they also assessed the volunteers for chronic disease risk factors.

Their conclusion: "This lifestyle modification program is an efficacious nutrition and physical activity intervention in the short term and has the potential to dramatically reduce the risks associated with chronic diseases in the long term."

In six weeks, those in the intervention group had chosen, because of the education they received, to increase their physical activity and to begin eating diets based on unrefined foods like whole grains, raw nuts, legumes, fresh fruits and vegetables.

The intervention group showed significant reductions in body fat, cholesterol levels and blood pressure, in addition to increased knowledge about how to sustain a healthy lifestyle.

Research studies of a control group of men and women aged 65 to 79 years, conducted by the Milia Kivipelto Aging Research Center in Sweden with results published in *Lancet Neurology* in October of 2005 has also shown that regular exercise (perhaps partly due to increased protein flow) reduces the risk of developing Alzheimer's by as much as sixty percent. Researchers also documented a significant improvement in cognitive ability in women who exercised regularly when they were between the ages of forty and sixty.

Physical exercise definitely supports brain health by increasing the delivery of oxygenated blood to every part of the body. This ensures that the chemical action nourishing existing brain cells aids in the formation of healthy new cells. While increasing blood flow, exercise also works to lower blood pressure. And high blood pressure presents a higher risk for memory loss.

Perhaps most heartening is the finding that, for those who have already contracted a degenerative disease like Alzheimer's, moderate exercise helps arrest, and can even reverse, the progress of the disease. As with other health aspects supporting the immune system, such as proper diet, exercise strengthens the immunity of the person who is ill. In so doing, it eliminates many of the conditions which helped breed the illness in the first place. It is vital that caregivers recognize the importance of exercise in assisting their patients and, within safe limitations, enjoy some form of movement with them every day.

Walk Away from Alzheimer's

So, are those who cannot afford gym memberships or exercise classes doomed to disease and early death? Of course not. We are also learning that easy, inexpensive and cost-free exercise, like walking, can have a phenomenally beneficial impact on health if done frequently and consistently.

Walk Your Body

The best way to make sure we get enough exercise, of course, is to set a schedule for it and stick to that schedule. The schedule or plan could be something as simple as forgoing one after-dinner sitcom on TV to go for a walk. Ten minutes out, ten minutes back, and the rest of the evening is all yours (and with VCRs, DVD recorders, and all the other recording means available, you don't even have to miss that program).

To avoid frustration, go for time and not distance. Walk at a pace that is comfortable for you. Begin walking for a length of time that you can manage. You will enjoy it, and with success, you will be encouraged to add on to your "out and back" time. Plan routes past scenes, such as parks or landmarks that you will enjoy; stroll past that house where there is a renovation going on, which you can't quite see as you zoom by in a car. You'll discover all sorts of sounds, smells, and textures when you walk through your world instead of driving past it.

Not the structured type? Does a daily walk still have that exercise class feeling for you? It is possible to incorporate walking into your daily life without very much disruption to your routine. It's easy when you look for opportunities to walk.

Take the stairs instead of the elevator. Instead of looking for the parking space closest to the door, park a few rows, or all the way, back.

There are many other ways to slip exercise into your life. Take your cue from the World War II era slogan, "Is this trip necessary?" Formulated to remind citizens to conserve fuel and oil, the phrase can still help us determine if we need to get into our vehicles. For example, do you have several errands that take you to the same general neighborhood? Is it really necessary to ease into traffic out of one parking lot, only to pull into another one a short distance away? Plan your route (pick up frozen or heavy items last), park once, and walk around to your locations. In no time, you can have the day's exercise—and your errands—all accomplished.

Are you near public transportation? Leave the car at home and let someone else drive you to work or shopping. It takes a certain amount of walking to get to the train, bus, or subway stop, and when you get to the mall or downtown shopping area, you will have no choice but to walk from shop to shop. At the least, you'll walk from your stop to your job, and getting off a stop or two before you need to will add up fast for your exercise quota. Walk back to your stop for the ride home and, once again, your exercising is accomplished. (By taking public transportation, you help reduce the amount of toxins in the air that break down cells and lead to disease, so you win twice.)

If you're still having trouble getting motivated, consider using the buddy system. Commitment to helping support someone else's health in addition to your own may be just what it takes to get you going—especially if he or she comes knocking on your door and says, "Let's go!"

Walk Your Mind

Of course, there are many exercises other than walking that are fun and still fairly simple and inexpensive. You may prefer them because they are not as boring to you, and instinctively, you are choosing activities that support brain health. Any activity that engages your brain stimulates the chemical activity that keeps it healthy. This could be playing shuffleboard, darts, chess, checkers, and the like, which require eye-hand coordination and decision-making, to volleyball, tennis, etc., which require strategizing and reacting to others in addition to those skills just mentioned.

Remember your walking buddy? Talk to him or her while you're walking. Your discussion stimulates your brain while the rest of your body is getting its workout.

If you're walking alone, sing a song, or recite poetry, or do multiplication tables in your head, anything to get your brain pumping along with your feet.

Is the best exercise for you found on equipment? Exercise your mind by reading while cycling or walking or running on apparatus that accommodates a book. If you're not trespassing in his or her zone, talk to your neighbor on the next piece of equipment.

A Little More Structure

Some of the patients treated at my organization's facilities suffered from mental, physical and emotional disorders. However, the treatment modalities at that time were limited. In my search to help these patients, in the early 1960's, I involved Joseph Pilates and Swami Yogi Vishnudevananda in developing programs to help these patients, overseen by the Anbar Institutes. Today, yoga practices are an integral part of medical programs from Harvard Medical School, Massachusetts General Hospital, UCLA and medical centers around the country specializing in reversing many chronic illnesses.

Dharma Singh Khalsa, M.D., president and medical director of Alzheimer's Prevention Foundation International, calls exercises such as these "brain aerobics," and he recommends them in his new work, *The Better Memory Kit: 7 Days to Better Memory.*

Dr. Khalsa recommends regular aerobic exercise and weight training (thirty minutes, three to four times per week), which can include something as simple as walking. To add the brain exercise component, Dr. Khalsa recommends exercises taught to him by Yogi Bhajan, whom he describes as a great yoga master of our generation.

Dr. Khalsa notes that at only three percent of our body weight, our brains receive, and require, a disproportionate amount—twenty-five percent— of the blood pumped by our hearts. Conditions that develop through the years, such as hardening of the arteries and high cholesterol, can appreciably reduce that blood flow.

In *The Better Memory Kit,* Dr. Khalsa recommends two simple yoga exercises, one that increases the blood flow to the brain, and one that sends direct healing energy there.

The CD that accompanies Dr. Khalsa's kit explains in full detail, but the simple, basic description should encourage you to try yoga, if you haven't yet experienced this form of mind/body exercise.

Exercise to Increase Blood Flow

Sit in a comfortable position on the floor or in a chair. Place your arms out to your sides and make your hands into a claw. Raise your arms, palms up, and then raise them higher up and cross them over your head, right over left and left over right. Repeat this motion breathing deeply and rhythmically. Continue for three minutes. Then, thrust out your tongue and continue the movement for 15 more seconds. Exhale, and repeat. Then, inhale again and hold the position for 15 seconds. Exhale and then use a relaxation exercise.

Kirtan Kriya

This exercise, whose name means a "singing exercise complete in itself," adds five ingredients to the four parts of basic meditation: comfort, quiet, a tool, and a special attitude, which says to start all over again when other thoughts enter your mind.

The five new ingredients added are:

1.   Breath

2.   Posture

3.   Healing sounds

4.   Fingertip position

5.   A unique focus of concentration

The exercise is also known as the five primal sounds meditation. The healing sounds are called primal sounds because, according to yogis, they are the five most healing sounds in the universe.

The four sounds are Sa, Ta, Na, and Ma. A fifth sound, Ah, is sounded at the end of the others, making five sounds in

all. Because the breathing is dictated by the sounds, it naturally is done correctly.

While chanting the sounds, the meditator touches the
thumb to the index finger, middle finger, ring finger, and pinky
finger in turn with each successive sound. Also while chanting,
the meditator imagines the sound entering the top of the head
and exiting through the forehead in an *L* meditation.

On the energy level, the sound opens a channel among the
top of the head, the seventh energy center of the body (which
corresponds to pineal gland) and the sixth energy center,
which corresponds to the pituitary gland.

There is also solid science behind the positive effect Kirtan
Kriya has on the brain. Management of the fingers occupies a
large portion of the brain, which is quite logical considering the
almost ceaseless activity of the fingers compared to other body
parts. Therefore, touching the fingers together energizes the
brain, while also inducing a relaxed state.

Singing or chanting the five primal sounds has a positive
effect on the chemistry of the brain. There are fifty-four
points, similar to acupuncture points, located on the upper
palate, the roof of the mouth. Directly on the other side of the
upper palate are the hypothalamus and pituitary glands, the
master glands of the brain.

During chanting, the tongue touches the roof of the mouth, and subtle energy in the form of sound vibrations move
through the palate to the pituitary gland. Then the pituitary
directs the release of healing chemicals that improve memory.
The beneficial effect continues as the chemicals are then trans-
ported by the bloodstream throughout the body.

Dr. Khalsa, who is also the author of *Brain Longevity,* began
his career as a researcher in the use of epidural anesthesia. His
observations during that time of the effects of stress on memory
coincided with his becoming acquainted with Yogi Bhajan.

Those two influences led Dr. Khalsa to search for solutions to the problem through integrative medicine, a field that combines traditional and complementary medical disciplines for the best result. Dr. Khalsa reports that researchers have documented positive changes in the brain following meditation. They have seen an unhealthy brain, with depressions and flatness that represent decreased flow of blood and energy, become plump and healthy looking after meditation.

To find a yoga book or recording that suits you, consult with your local librarian or the Internet. Churches, synagogues and civic groups such as the local YMCA, also offer programs if you would like to practice in a group. Consult your phone book or the community pages of your local newspaper to find a compatible group.

Chapter Five

A World Without Alzheimer's

"Strictly speaking, it is not normal to grow old. Health should be considered the norm."
Joseph W. Still

Painless movement. Boundless energy. Sharp perceptions and memory.

We in the western world leave some of these healthy conditions behind with our childhood, and we accept that the rest will vanish with age. We believe that to continue on in that healthy state would be nirvana—literally, a spiritual paradise separate from the body.

There are, as I have said previously, places in the world where people carry these healthy characteristics far into adulthood. I have already mentioned the Hunza, and we will now take a closer look at them, for we can obtain great insight and encouragement from their health; their untainted lifestyles can teach us much about achieving that same robust vitality.

67

Hunza

Shangri-La. Heaven on earth. It is no accident that author James Hilton chose the land on "the roof of the world" as the setting for *Lost Horizon*, his story of a fictional paradise whose inhabitants have eternal youth.

Here we find Hunza (pronounced Hoonza), a small town located high in the Hindu Kush Mountains in the northern part of the Indian subcontinent, where the borders of Kashmir, China, India, and Afghanistan meet. It is located on the banks of the river of the same name, and visitors must travel a mountain road from Gilgit to find it, surrounded by deep gorges and huge glaciers like the Ulter, watched over by the Himalayas, including the Rakaposhi (*Britannica* 2005).

Difficult as it is to travel to this region 9000 feet above sea level, the Hunza have played host to travelers on their way from the Hindu Kush to the Vale of Kashmir. Even though exposed to travelers from the outside, western world, the community has remained homogenous, and its customs have survived down through the ages.

The Hunza's obscure origins are rooted in myth and legend, which claim that they are descendents of deserters from the army of Alexander the Great, soldiers who fled with their Persian wives to the region around 300 B.C. (Godefroy 2001). They continued their military tradition for several centuries, raiding and plundering neighboring communities. After a time they became tillers of the soil, and their existence has been peaceful, if primitive, ever since.

Today they are subsistence farmers who do not engage in trade and do not possess any form of currency. Neither are they craftsmen, but they have developed irrigation systems, and raise cattle and cultivate crops of rice, maize (corn), fruits, and vegetables.

What some may see as a hard life (a hardy life would be a more apt description) is actually the key to the Hunzas' long and healthful existence. It is commonplace for a Hunza to live to be one hundred years old. In fact, many live to be 130, and there are reports of many living to the age of 145 (Godefroy 2001).

Where Disease Is a Stranger

First reports to the western world out of this mountaintop utopia came from a Scottish physician, Dr. Robert MacCarrisson, who spent seven years with the Hunza between the two world wars.

Dr. MacCarrisson reported that the Hunza were exceptionally vigorous and robust. He also noted that they suffered from none of our modern diseases. There was no evidence of cancer or heart disease, the two biggest killers in the West, or any of the lesser ailments such as arthritis, stomach ulcers, hypertension, diabetes, and varicosity.

Children were also disease-free and showed no signs of mumps, measles, chicken pox, or any of our usual childhood ailments. Infant mortality was also extremely rare.

Ageless Aging

MacCarrisson noted that not only were the Hunza not sick, they went about living their lives with a physical energy and mental enthusiasm that would be unheard-of in a westerner of the same advanced age. In a community where living through one century and well in to the next is the norm, attitudes about personal abilities are radically different from those of westerners. There are reports of eighty-year-old Hunza women working for hours on end at arduous physical tasks like chopping wood and moving rocks while showing very little fatigue.

Their appearance is ageless as they go about these youthful

activities. Climbing and descending steep mountainsides regularly leaves them lean and muscular, with straight posture and a graceful step. They have no experience of following specialized diets in order to lose weight; they do not have cellulite and would not even understand the concept.

Further reports state that it is quite normal for ninety-year-old Hunza men to father children. Witnesses also report seeing men over one hundred-years-old carrying heavy loads up the rocky mountain paths, becoming no more fatigued or out of breath than the average forty-year-old westerner.

A group of seventy-year-olds was observed by western visitors playing a game of volleyball which included a man more than twice their age (reportedly 145). The older man matched them spike for spike and jump for jump. Then, without resting, he went off to a meeting of elders located in a building on a cliff some 1,500 feet above the volleyball field.

Considering such facts, it is easy to see that a two-hour walk would be child's play for the average Hunza. The Hunza take these walks after lunch to relax and reward themselves for their labors—and then they return refreshed to a long afternoon of work.

Can this vigor and longevity be attributed solely to genetics, to the strong bloodlines of Alexander's warriors? The Hunza offer us many clues and a model for healthy living.

Nutrition Is The Primary Key

First, we have to wonder what fuels the Hunza through long days spent working on the mountainside, without benefit of motorized vehicles or equipment, without huge breakfast platters of eggs, sausage, and potatoes, followed at day's end by dinners featuring slabs of meat and potatoes smothered in butter and sour cream. The average westerner eats this and more to see him through a day that typically holds little or no physical exertion.

Contrary to Western notions, which see breakfast as the most important meal, the Hunza see benefit in a morning's work on an empty stomach. They rise early and begin their labors, not pausing until noon for their first of two meals, which consist primarily of whole grains.

Dr. MacCarrisson believed that the Hunza diet contributed significantly to the community's overall health. As director of nutrition research for the Research Fund Association in India, Dr. MacCarrisson tested his theory in the laboratory by feeding a different diet to each of three groups of mice.

The first group thrived on a diet consisting exclusively of Hunza food. Dr. MacCarrisson chose the diet of neighboring Kashmir for the second group of mice. They developed several diseases.

The third group fared the worst of all—on a diet from a supposedly advanced nation. Following a steady diet of typical British food, the mice in that group quickly fell ill with symptoms of neurasthenia, a condition resulting in chronic fatigue and behavioral disorders.

"You are what you eat." This has been the view of experts from Hippocrates to modern-day nutritionists. If we desire to be robust, vigorous, and disease-free long into our lives, we would do well to carefully scrutinize the Hunza diet.

There are two aspects to it: quantity and quality.

Not only do the Hunza eat but two meals per day, they eat nowhere near the amount of food that westerners do. Their land and climate are harsh, and their Spartan ways make the most of the resources available.

Their simple food is delicious, but the Hunza eat for sustenance rather than for pleasure. Contrast this with our western eating habits. We choose food for its taste and appearance, not its nutritional value, and we keep eating long after we have obtained all we need to support life.

Never really allowed to rest, our stomachs exhaust themselves processing the endless supply of food we stuff down our gullets. This affects our nervous systems, circulation, colon and blood sugar, and we can become fatigued, ill, or even depressed.

When considering our situation in this rational light, most will see that it is an unhealthy and unnatural way to live, and yet, in the moment, we gorge ourselves as usual. As a species, we are irrational and no longer follow our instincts; we follow our wishes.

As a further example of how far we have become estranged from nature and instinct, consider reports that long before the tsunami struck Asia early in 2005, the animals ran for higher ground. The humans, who were attuned only to knowledge they could gain through physical sensation (we have for too long worshipped at the altar of empiricism), went about their business as usual until it was too late and disaster struck.

Animals also give us a lesson in following our instincts when it comes to eating. Obesity is not a problem in the natural world (although diet-food for overfed domesticated animals is becoming a cottage industry), and the animal who is ill refrains from eating altogether.

Abstention is a part of the Hunza's eating habits as well, with regular fasts as part of their routine. What the Hunzas do eat is free of chemical additives, with fruits and most vegetables consumed raw. When vegetables are cooked, it is for a short time. Fruits and vegetables are chosen from the very best nutritional sources.

Although the Hunza eat a primarily vegetarian diet, they also consume mountain goat milk products (primarily yogurt), which contributes to health by replenishing intestinal flora. Meat is eaten infrequently, at rare special occasions like weddings and festivals, and is served in small portions that have been stewed for many hours. The meat of choice is usually chicken.

We can see how, free from the westerner's burden of continuous digestion and its resultant fatigue, the Hunza's body efficiently utilizes nutrition and calories and provides nearboundless energy for work and play. Again, compare this to the western experience of ceaseless digestion, compelled by gorging on not only too much food but also on the wrong types, especially highly-processed red meat. More than three hours are required for the stomach to properly digest a normal portion of meat, and very few of us are content with eating merely two or three ounces. Consider also that the sedentary lifestyle of the average westerner ensures the dangerous buildup of cholesterol and waste products from this never-ending process. And cholesterol is a prime factor in heart disease. While there are other factors at work, blocked arteries can be attributed in a large measure to eating too much meat.

A special treat for the Hunza is apricot pits, and they eat almonds whole or process it into oil. In fact, nuts are often the meat, so to speak, of the meal. Nuts such as walnuts, hazelnuts, almonds, or beechnuts may be mixed into a salad. This often is the entire meal, rather than the preliminary or appetizer that it would be in the West.

Westerners can adapt the Hunza diet to their use with some thought and creativity. A good place to start is with grains. One caution: it is of no benefit to increase the intake of grains if they are eaten in the form of leached-out, refined white flour, often known among nutritionists as "white death." To obtain the benefits, it is necessary that the grain be whole grain, which means the germ is still intact. This is where many nutrients, including all of the grain's vitamin E, are found.

Staff of Life

A major source of whole grain in the Hunza diet is chapatti bread. Just as their fruits and vegetables are eaten raw or prepared fresh for that meal, chapatti is prepared for each meal using fresh ingredients with no preservatives or chemicals.

Appearing regularly in a diet marked by frugality, the chapatti seems to play a major role in the Hunzas' extraordinary longevity and good health. Chapatti is available in some health food stores; it looks nothing like the bread we are accustomed to eating. However, its nutritional value is significant. Remember that choosing whole grain flour is essential: the recipe calls for a combination of wheat and buckwheat flour, but the bread can be made from any whole grain, including millet and barley.

Emulating the Hunzas' diet can take us a long way down the road to health and into robust old age. There are three key concepts to bear in mind:

- Frugality: Listen to your body and eat only what you truly need. Remember the energy of the Hunza as they go about their labor-filled days.

- Freshness: Eat fruit raw and vegetables raw or lightly steamed to retain their nutritional value. Avoid meat altogether, but if you cannot, then try to lower your consumption as much as you possibly can. Buy unpreserved bread such as chapatti from freshly ground whole grain flour.

- Fasting: Fasting, preferably for one day a week, is considered to help rid the body of toxins that contribute to poor health.

Key Two: Exercise

Carrying heavy loads up and down mountain trails all day and working the soil by hand is certainly more exercise than the westerner gets in his or her average day, or his or her average month for that matter. However, the Hunza see wisdom in adding exercise, including sports, to their regimen.

Clearly most of us are not inclined to become farmers on a mountaintop, nor is it necessary to do so, but we should pay close attention to the benefits that the Hunzas derive from their active and strenuous lifestyle.

Westerners can easily practice the Hunzas' favorite exercise: walking. The mountain people take a daily walk and regularly embark on extended hikes of 15 or 20 kilometers.

For us, a daily walk for an hour will provide a complete workout for our bodies, and our minds benefit from the exercise as well. There is no equipment involved, no cost, and it's simple to do.

In addition to the movement involved, walking gives us another benefit by getting us out in the fresh air. The Hunza exercise outside as often as possible in order to breathe in the clean invigorating mountain air. Volleyball and polo are very popular for this reason.

We in the West have access to many sports that will get us out and get us moving. Organizations abound for all ages, and those who need the motivation of scheduling can find whatever they need or want.

One organized activity that has translated quite well to the west is yoga. Still gaining in popularity, instruction for this ancient art is easy to find in most communities. Once learned, it can be practiced at home.

More simply, we can find what we need by starting right at home. This has the advantage of attracting family members into the healthy practice of exercise. Set up the volleyball/badminton net and have an ongoing family or neighborhood tournament. Walk around the croquet course for a bit every night. Get out the ball and glove and have a toss. The possibilities are limited only by your interests and imagination.

Work Steadily and Relax

The traffic. The job. The bills. Most of us wake up in the morning, take the mental equivalent of a deep breath, and plunge into the stress that they never left behind even in sleep. This is the life most of us know, and we cannot conceive of its being any different.

The danger to our health is that we do not realize the extent of the damage caused by stress. Stress is not just a small factor that makes most days serious and unpleasant. The exploding demand for coping drugs shows how badly our mental and emotional well-being is compromised by stress. Left unresolved, it often leads to nervous breakdown.

Stress also kills, and scientists have proven its link to heart attacks, something the Hunza do not experience. In fact the Hunza believe relaxation to be so important that they find time each day to pursue it through brief meditation sessions. The young also take part in meditation. Given the pressure on Western children from SATs, SOLs, GPAs, and the rest of the stressors of academia, there is a loud clear message of health for them from the Hunza as well.

Yoga instruction can introduce the westerner to relaxation techniques. There are many, so it is possible to find one that suits individual's needs and preferences. Books abound on the subject, and for those wishing to explore the technique on their own, many health care professionals are available who can teach a variety of relaxation techniques.

For starters, try taking a few minutes several times a day

and practice slow, deep breathing. Sit or stand quietly and notice how your body and mind recharge as the calming effect of the breathing takes over.

When you return to work, take a page from the Hunza book and work serenely. The Hunza work at a slow, steady pace that permits them to work long hours. The pace also reflects an attitude that prevents exhaustion.

As with eating, westerners would greatly benefit by returning to a more instinctual physical life in matters of exercise and stress-control. We can put our heads down, burst into the fray, and push and eat ourselves into coronaries. Or, we can listen to our bodies. They tell us in no uncertain language all we need to know, and if we do not listen, they will scream the message in the form of nervous breakdown or heart attack.

Key Three: It's All in the Mind

The 'age of plenitude' is what the Hunza call their older years, the years beyond age 80. It is what we paradoxically call the golden years, though our attitudes make clear that we do not believe this to be so. For the Hunza, these are the years of full bloom, the ripe years when the summit of life and wisdom are reached. To a very large degree it is their outlook and expectation of long life which causes it to be so. ("I think, therefore I am," said the philosopher Descartes.)

The Hunza do not retire. They continue their daily work and play for as long as possible, and that time is very long, nearly twice our own lifetimes.

In sharp contrast we in the West grow old and die at ages which would shock the Hunza, who would consider us to be barely past youth. More shocking still to them would be the infirmities, the pain and suffering we undergo during those years.

The difference between their healthy longevity and the

Western lack thereof lies, I believe, in our psychology. Hunza children have before them every day the example of lives lived vigorously all the way to advanced ages. The Western mind is permeated with the twin messages that life can be expected to end somewhere around age 70 and that old age is useless and ugly, only youth is worthwhile and beautiful.

Sadly enough, Westerners have been highly proficient at living down to these expectations. However, things may be slowly changing, as more people become aware that truncated, pain-filled lives are not necessarily the norm, and that the goal of living long, healthful, fulfilling lives is eminently within our reach.

Researchers recently announced that the human body has been scientifically adjudged to be capable of functioning effectively well past one hundred years of age. Yet, our experience falls far short of the scientific possibility.

The Hunza attitude— that each passing year should be celebrated for the wisdom and prowess it has added to an individual's life— is the key to achieving our own longevity. Imagine this: you are sitting at your desk, and you ask a passing coworker for some object you need, a pencil perhaps. Instead of handing it to you, he or she tosses it to you. Are you more likely to catch that pencil if you think you can ... or if you think you cannot?

This is how the mind affects the body, a case if ever there was one of mind over matter. For if we believe we are destined to deteriorate and die well short of a century, then that is exactly what will happen. On the other hand, what might happen if we adopt the Hunza attitude that age is wealth to be spent on joy? If we are not prepared to understand this instinctually, we have plenty of scientific data that can corroborate it intellectually.

So what are we waiting for? Instead of getting old, let's live to a ripe old age.

Chapter Six

Immersion in a Therapeutic Environment is the Key

"Why should you wait until you are faced with a life-threatening health crisis to want Health Excellence? For optimal health, you must consume a diet with a high-nutrient per calorie ratio."
—Dr. Joel Fuhrman, *Eat to Live*

For many of us, the message of Alzheimer's comes too late. We eat crazily and continuously, and lead frantic lifestyles that leave our cells unprotected from the assaults of free radicals. This lifestyle, coupled with factors such as trauma or genetic vulnerability, causes our cells to degenerate. Then we, or a loved one, develop Alzheimer's. What then? As we have noted in earlier chapters, it is the body that heals itself. There are substances and elements we can obtain from the outside such as health-specific, immunity-inducing food, and medicines that support the effort and alleviate suffering from symptoms. But ultimately the body has got to repair itself.

This process requires much more than the ingestion of helpful agents, however. We must give the body a chance to function properly by *not* doing things which interfere with the functioning. To accomplish this, it is logical to adopt measures which will prevent our becoming ill in the first place. So when sickness strikes, the first thing is to remove the causes of sickness.

Total Immersion: The Healing Experience

To give the body the best chance of healing itself, the affected person should be totally immersed in healthy practices in every aspect of daily life. There are two ways to accomplish this. Home caregivers can help the individual to develop and follow a healthy regimen, or residential therapeutic communities can give individuals support, not only from their caregivers but also from other residents who are undergoing an identical experience.

Whatever the choice, the program should follow the principles of nature (the natural human program) to maintain health and prevent disease. In an appropriate program, the affected individual will:

- take in proper food and all nutrients.

- avoid foods that are toxic.

- avoid environmental toxins.

- lower stress through meditation and other mind/body methods.

- obtain psychosocial therapeutic interaction (family and friends can contribute greatly here).

- participate in daily exercise.

- receive the benefit of advanced medical diagnostic systems.

- receive all needed pharmaceutical and medical treatments, whenever needed.

- acknowledge and develop your spirituality

Should you choose home care, there are a number of websites that can help you with the many aspects of your choice, from anticipating your loved one's needs and ways you can provide assistance to finding professionals to help you both. You may want to begin your search by visiting some of these sites: www.careguide.com, www.evercareconnections.com, and www.seniorresource.com.

There are innumerable residential facilities, with widely varying philosophies, for individuals afflicted with Alzheimer's. When choosing a residential facility, it is important to look for one that not only employs medicine to treat symptoms and alleviate suffering, but also supports health, and embraces the possibility of recovery by following the laws of nature.

Facilities I was involved in creating have sought for fifty years to bring the best of both worlds to the patient. While supporting the laws of nature, they employ eclectic and holistic techniques, including medication, surgery, psychological and nutrition counseling, and other advanced technologies whenever necessary. Their goal is not only to provide the highest level of medical care, but also to support the best possible quality of life for those who join their communities. This is accomplished by enhancing emotional, cognitive, and spiritual health in addition to addressing physical needs.

You Are What You Eat

Like all living things, human beings are programmed for eating in a way that supports our health. For tigers, meat-eating is part of their programming. It is necessary for their health, and they instinctively stalk and kill their prey. On the other hand, a cow is not programmed to eat meat and therefore does not seek it in nature. Man has interfered here, and caused the cow to eat products from other animals, notably waste products from chickens. There is widespread belief that the recent epidemic of "mad cow disease" is a direct result of feeding cows material they are not programmed to consume, a gross violation of nature's law requiring not to consume toxic substances. It is important to note that the poultry products must be altered and disguised before the cows will accept them.

Over the decades science has methodically proven that the laws of nature are the ultimate blueprint for our health. For example, after many years of research medical science has discovered that Hippocrates, the ancient Greek physician known as the father of medicine, was right in his statement that "food is your medicine." He believed in the natural healing process of good diet, fresh air, rest, and cleanliness. It has taken twenty-five centuries, but medical science has finally caught up with Hippocrates and knowledge that was available two and a half millennia ago.

It is impossible to fool Mother Nature. Proper eating creates and supports health, while improper eating causes disease. In order to be healthy, we must obtain all required nutrients, found mostly in fresh fruits, vegetables, legumes, seeds, nuts, and avoid toxin-producing foods. If we do not follow these principles, our immunity decreases and we become weakened and vulnerable to degenerative diseases. If we are already sick, we must immediately change our food habits and follow healthy principles.

A Healthy Food Plan

When seeking a residential facility, look for one where the residents obtain a great deal of vegetables and fruits every day. This ensures that they consume all the nutrients they need, as well as helping to remove toxins from their bodies. In this way, the facility provides the opportunity for residents to improve and recover. By so doing, it signals that it believes in the possibility of recovery and honors the right of every resident to enjoy the highest quality of life possible.

The home caregiver can take a cue from such residential programs by providing primarily raw vegetarian foods in a clean, non-processed state. In fact, science concurs that this message from Alzheimer's has significance for all degenerative diseases. An example is the successful recovery from heart disease by those following programs such as those developed by Dr. Dean Ornish. The laws of nature clearly resound in his regimen of low-fat meals, exercise, and stress management.

As I have indicated, a healthful, nutritious, toxin-destroying diet should consist largely of vegetables. In fact I recommend a vegetarian diet to everyone, but at least seventy-five percent of food intake should consist of raw fresh vegetables and fruits; let us repudiate once and for all the obsolescent FDA 'food pyramid' that has contributed so much to today's obesity problem among children, with its heavy over-emphasis on carbohydrates. Fruits and vegetables, especially the green vegetables like broccoli and asparagus, even a baked potato, along with whole-grain foods will provide ample carbohydrates, and of the perfect type, containing natural sugars in moderate amounts that will not spike blood-sugar levels and wreak havoc on insulin production, which is a contributor to diabetes. They are also wonderful antioxidants. Given our current American diets, it is no coincidence that juvenile diabetes has reached unprecedented levels in recent years. And contrary to popular belief, you can obtain all the protein you need from vegetable, fruit, and grain sources. Here are some helpful hints from noted nutrition expert Dr. Lorraine Day, another amazing person who cured herself of cancer through a healthy diet, for maximizing their value in your own diet:

1. Try not to eat fruits with other foods at the same time. The fruit is digested more rapidly and nothing will be emptied into the intestine until the all other foods are digested.

2. Be sure to thoroughly chew. If not, food will not mix properly with salivary enzymes and will not digest properly. Also, inadequate chewing causes many nutrients to be lost.

3. In place of butter, you can use a little flaxseed oil and fresh lemon juice, which together look and taste like butter. Flaxseed oil is yellow; it is readily available in health food stores. It contains essential omega oils that cannot be produced by the body. However, it must be refrigerated before and after opening, and should never be heated or used for cooking.

4. Pasta, unless of the whole grain variety, should be shunned. It is nothing but paste—merely flour and water. It has virtually no food value and is simply empty sugar calories.

5. Eat very little bread, as it is a processed food high in calories and sugar. And eat only the whole-grain varieties which contain more nutrients and fiber. By contrast, white bread contains nothing of value and is laced with sugars, chemicals, and calories.

Chapter Seven

Early Detection: The Key to Defense

Imagine for a moment that you're experiencing symptoms such as memory loss, having to re-ask questions, and an inability to concentrate. Is this just normal aging, or the early signs of degenerative disease? Should you just shrug it off to having had a few too many birthdays? Or is Alzheimer's beginning its slow, unstoppable takeover of your brain?

With normal aging comes some degree of slowness, which also affects the memory. But troublesome signs—losing your way driving on familiar streets, or finding your car keys in improper places, call for a comprehensive evaluation, involving testing procedures administered by a competent physician.

That's important for two reasons: one, if you have the disease, early detection is vital; and two, certain disorders—depression, a blow to the head, or a thyroid problem, for instance—mimic the early signs of Alzheimer's. These ailments are eminently treatable and have much more predictable outcomes than a verdict of Alzheimer's.

The Preliminary Diagnosis

The so-called preliminary diagnosis is intended to rule out other possible causes of your symptoms. During your examination, it is important to ask your doctor questions, such as:

- What exactly does this diagnosis mean? If you don't fully understand what the doctor has found, ask him or her to explain it to you.

- Should I undergo more tests in order to confirm or dispute this diagnosis? Is there another doctor to whom I could be referred, if I so choose?

- What changes in behavior and mental ability am I to expect over a period of time?

- What care and treatments will I need?

- What can I do to alleviate the symptomatic problems?

Your doctor will also ask you questions about:

- **Medicines You're Taking.** Sometimes prescriptions (and even herbal remedies and over-the-counter aids) can interfere with each other, causing Alzheimer-like symptoms. Give your doctor a complete rundown of your drug intake.

- **What You're Eating and Drinking.** Nutrient-poor, neglectful meals can cause deficiencies that manifest in confusion, dizziness or incoherence—which mimic the classic early warning signs of Alzheimer's. Not taking in enough fluids (leading to dehydration) and alcohol abuse are two more bad habits that can act like early signs of the disease. Again, your doctor needs to know everything

about you in order to give you a truthful assessment of your condition; don't keep anything
inside.

- **Whether You Are Experiencing Lack of Sleep
  Due to Insomnia.**

One of the many helpful programs offered by The Alzheimer's Association is a two-hour workshop that will help you
make the most of your medical visits. Entitled "Partnering
with Your Doctor," Association representatives offer strategies
and resources that will help to improve communication with
your doctor. For anyone with the disease, as well as for those
who will be caring for the patient as time goes by, these work-
shops are invaluable.

Action Strategies

If the preliminary diagnosis, follow-up examination (second
opinion) and tests confirm the presence of Alzheimer's, your
immediate reaction will no doubt be one of sadness, anxiety and
fear. This is completely understandable. But, it's also urgent that
you, your loved ones and your physician or specialist begin to formulate a plan of action to cope with this disease, seek available
solutions and to try to keep it from worsening.

The years ahead will be a difficult challenge for you as well as
your family, but there are definite strategies available. One is seeking help from the Alzheimer's Association— it offers educational
and support programs for patients and their families, and keeps
up with the latest available treatment opportunities and research
in the field. With a national network of 81 chapters and 300 local
points of service, the Association's trained staff offers one-on-one
assistance and vital help to the 5 million Americans afflicted with
this disease.

Remember, too, that not only is help available today, but research in finding prevention and cure has never been more promising. William Thies, vice president of the Alzheimer's Association, predicted in early 2005 that screen tests, routinely administered once you reach age 55, would become reality in his lifetime. (Dr. Theis was 63 at the time). Such tests would suggest the beginning of treatment and prevention, even before the first symptoms appeared.

Positive Thinking: Your Strongest Ally

Striving for the highest quality of life in this difficult time and seeing every day as a new challenge are two major strategic elements in overcoming the obstacles of Alzheimer's. To achieve these goals, you must team up with your doctor and your family to form a unified front against this disease. You and your family must begin to educate yourselves, make important changes, and come to decisions in your life that may critically affect your future and avoid the progression of the illness.

All family members are an integral part of the treatment team, with specific duties and responsibilities that are part of the overall strategy. For example, the doctor will monitor your condition over time with brain scans and other tests that measure your cognitive functioning. That's the doctor's job. Your job is to stay active and informed, follow proper diet as instructed and take your medications if needed. It is essential to tell your doctor of any changes in your condition as soon as possible. This is one example of how you and your doctor can work together to further your overall strategy.

Prescription Drugs in Conventional Treatment

Researchers have developed two classes of FDA-approved

drugs for the treatment of the cognitive symptoms of Alzheimer's disease: Cholinesterase Inhibitors and Memantine (Approved by the FDA for Alzheimer's treatment in 2003). Cholinesterase inhibitors prevent the breakdown of acetylcholine, a chemical messenger in the brain that affects memory and thinking skills. About half of all patients who take this drug have shown a modest improvement in cognitive ability. The three most commonly prescribed medications in this class are: Aricept (Test results published in Journal of the American Medical Association after the Peterson study conducted at the Mayo Clinic), Exelon ("Staying Connected," Exelon internet website), and Razadyne (Johnson & Johnson Press release in 2005 stated that the drug containing the active ingredient galantamine, delays symptoms of memory loss and cognitive impairment). Cognex, approved in 1993, was the first cholinesterase inhibitor, but is rarely used today because of adverse side effects such as liver damage.

Memantine goes under the trade name Namenda. It was approved in 2003 for the treatment of moderate to severe dementia resulting from Alzheimer's disease. This drug, which comes in tablet form, seems to help regulate glutamate, a messenger chemical responsible for processing, storing, and retrieving information in brain cells. Excessive amounts of glutamate can lead to the destruction of brain cells.

Alternative Natural Nutrients

There is growing evidence that certain compounds, found primarily in healthful foods, can help prevent and alleviate Alzheimer's. For example, vitamin E, found in spinach, broccoli, nuts, and certain fruits and oils, may help prevent damage to brain cells caused by "oxidative stress" from so-called free radicals—molecules in our blood. However, research on vitamin E supplements in isolation has shown mixed results that are still being evaluated.

Ginkgo Biloba is said to have positive effects on both the brain and the body because of its antioxidant and anti-inflammatory properties. It is also known to protect cell membranes, and regulate neurotransmitter function. Thus, it is being used widely in Europe as a remedy for cognitive dysfunction. Although few side effects are associated with excessive Ginkgo Biloba, research studies such as one conducted by Pierre L. Le Bars, M.D., Ph.D., of the New York Institute for Medical Research, found no significant difference in overall impairment by taking Ginkgo biloba. However, the results did show enough improvement in cognition during daily activities and social interaction to warrant additional research in order to determine exactly how it works and the extent of its effect.

GETO, a Chinese herbal extract, also shows promise in treating Alzheimer's patients. This substance has been used to correct memory problems in China for centuries. Dr. Jinzhou Tian of the Dongzhimen Hospital at Beijing University of Chinese Medicine reported that patients with Mild Cognitive Impairment (MCI) who took GETO for three months showed improved cognitive function. Larger studies are now being planned.

Evaluating the Benefits

Because medicine is an art, and not an exact science, drug therapy is not guaranteed to provide instant or even reliable results. You and your doctor can determine if a drug is helping you, or whether you might need a different drug or a different dosage. Some prescriptions work well on one patient but do not work as well on another. Also, if you have any side effects or adverse effects from a drug, which happens often, report it to your physician immediately in order to prevent further damage.

You should be in constant communication with your doctor. Only then can you both formulate the best plan for your treatment. Keep the following questions in mind when you visit with or speak to your doctor:

- How do you measure if a drug is working?
- How much time has to pass before we know if a drug is effective?
- How will you monitor for side effects of the drug?
- What are the symptoms of side effects that I should be concerned about?
- Is any one drug more likely to interfere with other medications or conditions?
- Is it dangerous to switch medications?
- Will I ever be able to stop taking the medication?

Should You Enter a Clinical Trial?

You may also want to consult your physician about participating in a clinical trial for experimental drugs. Pharmaceutical companies, the U.S. federal government, and the Alzheimer's Association all fund research studies to learn about the disease, to relieve symptoms, and to stop the disease from occurring.

Clinical trials test the safety and efficacy of new drugs before the FDA approves them. If you are interested in participating in a clinical study, the Alzheimer's Association can provide information about such studies being conducted near your home. If you decide to participate, you may need to answer additional questions and take additional tests. There is a large time commitment on your and your family's part as well. Finally, it is important to be aware of the risk involved in this process because the drug you may take is still in the experimental stage.

Keeping Your Family Close

Never be afraid to discuss your condition with your family because you will need and want their support. Explaining the condition to them will alleviate their anxiety and help them work with you to formulate the best possible plan to cope with the coming years. Both you and your family must consider many factors, including finding out all about the disease and its various treatment possibilities, to halting degeneration, creating the best environment possible and seeking the best future care for improvement. This is important, not only for your own care, but also for the family's knowledge to help their own prevention. By doing so, you are actually helping them as well.

You may also want to discuss various legal and financial aspects of your situation, as well as thinking about advanced directives. The more communication there is early on, the more positive the results may be. Now is the time for everyone to pull together and fight hard against the enemy, which is Alzheimer's disease.

It is important for you to keep as active as possible or even to increase your mental and physical activities as much as possible. Activities stimulate brain cells to grow, so now is not the time to give up and lie around the house alone. You should continue to see friends and family, and participate in social and religious activities. A program of light aerobics such as walking and swimming would be ideal for you. If you have any hobbies or interests, try to continue them if at all possible, or develop new interests. Reading is also a valuable exercise that stimulates the brain, as are singing, listening to music, and dancing.

On the Horizon: Promising Research

The trend in Alzheimer's research now is going from drugs that merely relieve symptoms to treating the underlying causes of the disease. As mentioned already, there has never been a more promising time for researchers looking to unlock the mysteries of Alzheimer's. Many of the studies underway today have begun to examine the brain's chemical processes, in hopes of identifying and containing harmful compounds that interrupt its normal functions.

One accepted explanation for how Alzheimer's develops is known as the Amyloid Hypothesis. This theory says that a chemical process causes strands of amyloid beta peptides to accumulate on the tissues of the brain, eventually forming plaques that disrupt communication between brain cells, causing cell death. Alzheimer's patients have much more of this protein than do normal persons.

However, several new treatment methods are targeting beta amyloid. Various theories about the connection between amyloids and brain cell death are now being thoroughly tested; if successful, this research may someday lead to better treatments, or even a cure.

In one study, Dr. Marc Weksler, Wright Professor of Medicine at the Memory Disorders Program at the Weill Medical College of Cornell University, explored the use of immunoglobulin (IVIg) on eight patients with mild to moderate Alzheimer's disease. IVIg is derived from human blood and contains high concentrations of antibodies, including antibodies to beta amyloid. After treating these patients for six months, Dr. Weksler observed a 45 percent decrease in beta amyloids, and six out of the eight patients had greater cognitive function. This is not available as a treatment, but more research on immunoglobulin influence on Alzheimer's will be further studied among larger clinical trials.

Researchers at the University of Bristol's Dementia Research Group in Great Britain have reported modestly encouraging results with Flurizan (This drug has completed a phase two clinical trial in 207 Alzheimer's patients; Stockholm Sweden in 2005). Although the results on the 207 participants were not statistically significant, the patients taking this drug did better than the placebo group in cognitive tests, including thinking and memory, and functioning in everyday life. However, those with mild Alzheimer's who received high doses did receive statistically significant results on cognitive test scores.

Lack of insulin productivity has been associated with Alzheimer's disease. Researchers from the University of Washington School of Medicine and the Veterans Affairs Sound Medical Center reported the results of testing the administration of intranasal insulin on early Alzheimer's patients. Their results showed that such administration might benefit patients with abnormal insulin regulation. The study also showed that Alzheimer's patients metabolize insulin differently. Further, this leads to the possibility of using other peptide substances in a similar way.

Experimental trials are underway for a drug called Alzehemed (FDA approved for Alzheimer's treatment in Wyeth Inc. and Elan Corp. study in 2004). This drug appears to bind to the chemical that forms clumps of plaque in the brain (beta-amyloids) and filter them out of the body. Alzehemed has shown significant progress in patients with mild Alzheimer's so far, and if subsequent clinical trials are successful, it could be on the market within the next five years.

In another area of research, scientists are now testing a biologically engineered version of an amyloid antibody. Since Alzheimer's patients have lower levels of such antibodies, this could prove to be a huge breakthrough in reversing the effects of the disease.

Other research is underway to develop a drug that blocks the production of the kind of beta amyloids which appear to cause Alzheimer's, without blocking the beneficial types, which are needed by the body. Still other researchers are experimenting with hormones, instead of chemicals, to block amyloid production.

Another therapeutic approach comes from Dr. Mark Tusznski of the University of California, San Diego. He has injected the brains of eight patients with specially engineered skin cells that work as tiny pumps that produce chemicals involved in nerve growth to prevent the withering away of brain cells. Almost two years later, there was a reduction of disease progression in patients with Alzheimer's by 36 to 51 percent, and there was an increase in normal activity on PET scans compared to untreated patients.

What About Stem Cell Research?

Stem cell research is a relatively new area of scientific research, and may be beneficial in preventing, treating, and even curing Alzheimer's disease one day.

There are two different types of stem cells: adult and embryonic. Stem cells can divide and replenish other cells such as muscle, blood, and brain cells. Embryonic stem cells have been fertilized in a woman's body and donated, and/or can be produced in the laboratory. These types of stem cells can theoretically turn into any type of cells in the body. While this type of research potentially holds great promise for some, there is also much opposition to using embryonic stem cells based on ethical and religious beliefs.

Stem cell research presently holds for some scientists the greatest promise for dealing with conditions such as Juvenile

Diabetes, Parkinson's disease, and spinal cord injuries. However, the mechanisms of Alzheimer's and the many brain cells involved make the use of stem cells very problematic. In fact, a host of medical experts see Alzheimer's not as a cellular disorder, but as a "whole brain disease."

The Internet and Alzheimer's

The Internet is a valuable resource for Alzheimer's patients and their families—one that wasn't even available to them a decade ago. Not only can patients find the latest information about the disease, the latest treatment strategies, new research, and other news, but they can also use it to join a support group. This ability to connect with information and people quickly can go a long way toward alleviating the anxiety and depression that patients and families often face. The Internet is home to a vast network of professionals, patients, and caregivers who are more than willing to share valuable information as well as the support patients and families need.

One group worth noting is the Center for Aging Services Technologies (CAST), an Internet organization that is constantly working to improve the care and services for Alzheimer's patients. CAST members are concerned with developing technologies that will allow patients to remain independent; allow professionals to obtain needed information more quickly; improve the communication links between patients and their families with service providers; and provide access to services that are far away. This is referred to as "enabling" technology.

Operational technology is useful to staff involved with Alzheimer's patients. Now, through the use of technology, they can participate in seminars and in-service training from various locations. This keeps staff up to date on all aspects of dealing with the disease.

Connective technologies allow communication between patients, caregivers, and support personnel. Thus, they can get answers, and often assistance, via the telephone and/or the Internet.

Telemedicine may prove beneficial to Alzheimer's patients, especially if they live alone. While now in the experimental stage, it has the potential of monitoring activities such as sleeping, eating, and taking medications.

Certainly, the Internet has changed the world, and makes it a smaller and friendlier place. If used wisely, patients and their families can find a great deal of comfort in this new technology. Not only can they find valuable information, which can empower them in their struggle, but they can meet new friends who make the fight and the journey a little easier to cope with. Your world can now actually expand instead of decrease because you can access people all over the world who share a common experience and a common goal. This could be a very exciting adventure for you, and you may learn new things every day, as well as making many new friends.

So, now that you have read all of this, try not to be overwhelmed by your mission, which is to try to save your brain. Basically, it boils down to several things:

Make sure that your diagnosis is correct.

- Discuss your condition with your physician and your family and formulate a plan of action.

- Follow your doctor's instructions, and report any problems to him immediately.

- Keep as active and positive as possible. Continue your routines, and be determined to learn new things.

- Learn to use technology to your benefit. The

Internet will open a whole new world to you—a world of knowledge and new friends.

• Know that you are not alone in your fight.

The Alzheimer's Association has joined with over 150 local, state, and government organizations representing 50 million people for the Coalition of Hope. So, clearly, you are not alone in your fight!

The knowledge that you gain along the way can be passed along to others as well and, therefore, will become part of the intensive research and data collection on Alzheimer's disease. Therefore, you should perhaps keep a diary of your activities and your thoughts. You are living at the most exciting time in medical and scientific research — a time when we may actually see a cure and/or prevention for Alzheimer's within our lifetime.

A Safe Place for Patients

One way of defending against Alzheimer's-related mishaps is to make sure that your home is safe. This "safe house" concept is, essentially, a house that has devices to help patients remain independent. For example, it comes with "artificial intelligence" to shut down stoves and remind them to take their medications on time.

With proper care and treatment, patients can continue living at home if they don't have a better alternative, which exists. In fact, according to the Alzheimer's Association, more than 7 out of 10 patients continue to live at home and receive care from family and friends. However, it is important to make the home environment as safe as possible. It should go without saying that a home with an Alzheimer's patient must be organized and free of clutter to make daily life go as smoothly as possible. The family should get together in order to make an assessment of any changes or improvements that have to be made.

There is much interest in architectural design to accommodate Alzheimer's patients, and it has been widely written about in aging and health care literature. An article in Human Ecology describes how students designed housing for Alzheimer's patients in order to provide safe and comfortable living arrangements for them. The students came up with unique design ideas for Shared Journeys, a New York City based organization involved in developing assisted living units for Alzheimer's patients. Some of the ideas involved kitchen cabinets with see-through fronts and large knobs, while other cabinets designed for caregivers had safety latches and held sharper objects that could be dangerous to an Alzheimer's patient. Bathtubs came with cascading water instead of a conventional faucet, and also with seats built in for the patient and caregiver. Medicine cabinets were locked, and the light source was incandescent instead of harsh and glaring.

There are many other things to do to avoid confusion and disorientation:

- Extra light should be provided in areas such as hallways, bathrooms, outside landings, stairways, entries, and areas between rooms.

- Area rugs of different colors should be placed by staircases, room entrances, and doorways to help differentiate that the environment is changing.

- Water temperatures should be monitored to avoid burns because the patient may become less sensitive to temperature changes.

- Grab-bars should be installed in bathrooms and showers along with non-slip surfaces in shower stalls.

- Use of appliances such as lawn mowers, mixers, grills, and knives should be limited and only conducted when someone else is present.

- Smoking and drinking alcohol should be monitored carefully.

- Objects such as magazine racks, coffee tables, and floor lamps should be removed to prevent falls for a person with limited concentration who may be wandering.

- Clean out the refrigerator at regular intervals in order to discard spoiled foods.

- Always lock up all firearms or remove them completely.

- Avoid slippery surfaces on all floors, and avoid busy patterns on floors and furniture.

- There should be a contrasting color between the floor and the furniture.

- Avoid clutter on the floor and around the room.

- If necessary, install an alarm system to avoid wandering outside, which could be dangerous.

- Always keep working fire extinguishers around the home.

- Keep emergency numbers available for the police, fire departments, and physicians.

Because these changes to the home are not that difficult to accomplish, the Alzheimer's patient may be able to remain at home for many years. These changes or accommodations do not need to be installed all at the same time, but can be phased in as necessitated by the individual patient's needs.

Patients who are at risk for getting lost outside of the home because of memory lapses can enroll in a program called Safe Return run by the Alzheimer's Association. This is a nationwide program that can identify, locate and return patients who have wandered off and do not remember how to get home again.

All this provides a certain degree of safety for the patient, but it doesn't facilitate improvement or an opportunity for reversing the disorder.

Holistic Solution

At the present time, there are two ways to approach the Alzheimer's problem. One is the conventional way, which means accepting the disease as incurable at the present time because there isn't yet a curable drug, hence waiting until a miracle drug will be developed. In the meantime, just find ways to keep the deteriorating person safe and learn about the interactive problems as much as possible. This is one approach to a solution.

The second approach is a natural holistic solution. This approach is based on considering life and health as part of nature. This approach perceives nature from a holistic viewpoint, which is completely interactive. Nature has its structure and laws, and any interference and intervention can cause damage both in the external or internal environment. Therefore, in order to prevent damage (disease), it is essential to follow these laws of nature and, in order to recover from a disease, it is necessary to return to the laws of nature. In order to maintain health, we need to know what these laws are, otherwise we cannot follow them unless we live in a community and environment where everyone follows these laws and no one lives differently. In the past few years, many scientific studies indicate that these laws have a lot of merit. For example:

A   Interference with the ecological environment causes pollution of the air and water, as well as global warming, which causes sickness to all animals, including human beings.

B   Artificial changes in agriculture and the use of chemicals, pesticides and genetic manipulations have proven to be harmful to both human beings and animals. As a result, there is now a trend to go back to natural produce now called "organic."

The same thing occurs in our internal diseases. If we interfere and intervene with the laws of nature, which created us, we cause harm to ourselves and become sick and die prematurely. This was well said by astronomer Carl Sagan: "Human misery is more often caused not so much by stupidity as by ignorance, particularly our own ignorance about ourselves."

If the damage already occurred, and we have become sick, should we wait ignorantly and passively for hopeful solutions to come from outside or should we seek to learn what the laws of nature are and be responsible for our own health? Naturally, the latter is the right answer. A person afflicted by Alzheimer's already cannot make the choice of seeking a solution on his or her own. The family must do it for them. There is hardly a chance for a patient to improve or even recover while staying at home because none of the causes of the disease are being removed. The only chance for improvement and recovery is to be immersed in a therapeutic environment where all causes known at present are being removed and do not exist. Such a therapeutic environment should provide the residents with:

1.   Organic food, which has all the required nutrients in the form of liquids and easily digested foods.

2.   Prevention of toxic food, water and air.

3.   Sufficient daily exercises for the body.

4.   Sufficient daily exercises for the mind.

5.   A great deal of social interaction.

6.   A secured environment without interfering with freedom of movement.

7.   Therapeutic activities for stress reduction.

8.   Opportunities for spiritual growth

All these can be provided only in a specialized environmental community. Without being in such a therapeutic environment, one cannot have the optimum opportunity or chance to improve or recover. The earlier a person with Alzheimer's is immersed in such an environment, the better the chance to improve and recover.

A solution to humans' problems cannot be found in the isolated details of the damages because humans are part of nature as a whole, governed by the laws of nature, and therefore can maintain our health and well being only by following these laws. We have to look at the whole picture and not pragmatically at a few isolated details because there is no end to the number of details, and we could never be able to identify them all because they run into the billions and trillions. Therefore, we have to follow the understanding of Albert Einstein who said, "Everyone who is seriously involved in the pursuit of science becomes convinced that a spirit is manifested in the laws of the universe — a spirit drastically superior to that of man."

Chapter Eight

A Family's Participation in Proper Care
Promotes Prevention for Its Own Members

By discovering the path to follow for preventing, lessening, or reversing Alzheimer's, patients' families help not only the patient but, equally important, themselves. They can use every bit of help available. Today there are about 20 million caregivers supporting 5 million Alzheimer's patients, and these numbers are rising rapidly; therefore any acquisition of knowledge and assistance for patients and their families is a tremendous boon to the entire country both health-wise and economically.

Dr. Abram Hoffer, the famous orthomolecular psychiatrist, said, "If you have only five minutes of lucid thought, Alzheimer's is reversible." As we have seen, the key lies in living the proper lifestyle. For both prevention of future disease and helping the patient already afflicted, the correct diet, nutritional supplements, exercise (physical and mental), and the reduction of stress are essential. If this is not possible in a home environment, which is often the case, it should be done in a specialized therapeutic community.

The best program for family members, as for all those intellectually able to choose a lifestyle, is to begin eating the right foods and taking proper supplements from the beginning. Just as family members help their ill loved ones to follow correct paths, they can also start themselves and their children on the right foods before children succumb to the blandishments of advertising and learn to do their own shopping. Parents must be acutely aware of the impact television ads that promote sugar/salt—coated products, fast food, have on children' s demands for such products. It is crucial to stimulate an early liking of nutritious foods. Parents thus give children a gift of love that will remain with them for a lifetime.

Since conventional medicine at the present time relies mostly on drug treatment of symptoms rather than removing the root causes of diseases, it will never succeed in curing most degenerative illnesses. Pharmaceutical researchers often promise that they are very close to developing a new drug that will cure a degenerative disease, but so far this has not occurred. For many years companies have attempted to develop and market wonder drugs to cure everything from cancer and cardiovascular disease to AIDS; yet the number of people suffering from these diseases has swollen to epidemic proportions. The truth is that no drug in isolation can cure degenerative diseases, including Alzheimer's. A drug at times may help, *but only if it is used in conjunction with a change in lifestyle.* It is tragic that so many people die each year because they rely solely on what is offered conventionally. They don't realize the simple truth: they need healthy living in all aspects of life. Why expect a change in results when there is no change in lifestyle choices?

Equally tragic is the fact that once the ravages of Alzheimer's have taken their toll, patients can no longer decide for themselves to initiate life changes; family, friends, or caregivers must do it for them. Additionally, since the disease causes problematic family and social interactions, it is often impossible to introduce the required changes at home to improve or even reverse the condition; the best solution, then, is to place the patient in a specialized therapeutic community where a healthy lifestyle is the only one available. In our culture, many people devour books and articles on staying healthy and eagerly watch news programs on health issues, but don't often put the ideas into practice. Remaining healthy is a day-to-day process of life, not just a once-in-a-while afterthought. It is as much a journey as a destination. A healthy body and mind make for a happier, fuller, richer, and ultimately longer, existence. This principle has been known throughout history. We can first practice healthy ways and then learn the reasons why these ways are necessary. As we discussed earlier, the Hunzas never read anything about health, but they practice healthy living. Learning is a wonderful tool, but our bodies are protected only when the learning is applied.

Now, there are always skeptics who will want more scientific proof before embarking on a healthy lifestyle. Junk-food advertisers spend billions trying to convince us to buy their products, but who is there to cajole us into eating a carrot? We ourselves must make choices we know are best for health. There are multitudes of testimonial accounts from people who have always lived healthily, and feel youthful, vigorous, and alert in later years, creating, working, traveling, participating in sports or music or art, or writing. They inspire others with their stories of the benefits of natural diet, supplements, exercise, and stress reduction. Some of the products known to be the most beneficial are the Vitamin B complexes, Vitamins A, D, E, and C, Ginkgo biloba, Gotu kola, Omega-3, Coenzyme Q-10, Ginseng, and even the spice, Rosemary. Many vitamin supplements now have high-performance ingredients which include these protective substances. Equally important is to eat a diet that includes fresh fruits and vegetables, oatmeal, seeds, nuts, oils, and fiber, which cleanse and help purify. Also, it is clear that optimum health requires avoiding, or at least lessening, meat consumption, and substituting high-protein alternatives. If children are offered only healthy foods, that is what they will learn to enjoy. The social value of eating these foods together as a family should not be underestimated. These behaviors not only protect the next generation, but are also critical components of helping a loved one with Alzheimer's. And good results will become readily apparent.

However, there are some who won't make life changes based only on the accounts of others. As I mentioned, they look for scientific data and formal studies. As yet there are virtually no studies detailing the significant role lifestyle plays in treating and controlling Alzheimer's disease, although the reality of many patients' lives has proven its importance. Fortunately, this may be about to change, as certain preventative measures are currently under study (more on these will be discussed in the next chapter). At a world conference on Alzheimer's in June, 2005, exciting evidence was presented identifying lifestyle as a major factor in any treatment program. However, it is not difficult to see why more studies have not been commissioned to date. Medical studies cost a great deal of money. Since most are funded by pharmaceutical companies, it is akin to expecting an oil company to conduct a study proving that solar energy is superior to gasoline. There is simply no incentive. But it is worth remembering that many, if not most, advances in the human condition have been made by individuals over the centuries without benefit of corporately-funded studies and elaborate symposia, often against furious, official opposition. Here are some encouraging examples to consider:

1. Two thousand years ago Hippocrates stated that "food is our medicine." He understood this long before scientists discovered the existence of vitamins, minerals, and proteins. He also realized the importance of rest, cleanliness, exercise and fresh air, and prescribed them for his patients.

2. Louis Pasteur discovered the role of bacteria and viruses in causing disease long before this was proven and accepted by the scientific community.

3. Kellogg founded Battle Creek Sanitarium, made famous in the movie, *The Road to Wellville*. He recognized the importance of fiber, a vegetarian diet, and the need for substantial fluid intake, prior to their value being demonstrated by scientific experimentation.

4. Einstein was fully aware of the splitting of atoms decades before it actually happened.

5. The writings of Freud and Jung and their documenting of unconscious complexes and processes were scoffed at by the scientific community (they became pariahs) for years before their theories were borne out in psychoanalytic practice.

Health based on the laws of nature has been understood in a variety of ways since time immemorial. Nowadays incorrectly called "alternative medicine," in reality it is caring for one's body by establishing healthy living habits, and is really not an alternative. Its growing popularity is directly proportionate to conventional medicine's failure to cure chronic and degenerative diseases. Lack of results is now forcing many physicians to learn about natural supplementation and begin to consider the merits of unconventional treatments, starting with a truly healthful diet.

Unfortunately, many current drugs *have proven* hazardous to our health in one way or another. It is just a matter of time for changes to occur. Natural supplements have had much less publicity, but the ideas of eating well, exercising, and keeping an active mind are beginning to spread throughout all segments of society.

We have already learned to our dismay that many drugs possess toxic side effects, and that these so-called "cures" are sometimes worse than the disease. This is an example of the law of unintended consequences. The much-hyped "wonder drug" for fertility of the late 1950s, thalidomide, caused thousands of children conceived from it to be born with abnormal or missing limbs. The point is that if we want to maintain good health, or if we are already sick and wish to recover, we should follow the basic principles of health that have existed for centuries, without passively waiting for miracles from the outside. After all, we are the ones living in our own bodies.

Now is the perfect time to seek healthy ways to prevent Alzheimer's, because in the twenty-first century, more doctors, scientists, and resources are devoted to the problem, and a new understanding of nature's curative power is beginning to emerge. Previously it was assumed that people who grew old were inevitably going to become forgetful. It was known as creeping senility. Now, since it has been recognized as a disease, there is world-wide interest. As I mentioned, in June of 2005, The Alzheimer's Association had its first International Conference on the Prevention of Dementia in Washington, D.C. About a thousand clinicians, researchers, and policy advocates from around the world discussed and explored new ways to prevent, diagnose, and treat this dreaded disease. Although there was much interest in new scientific research and technology, the "buzz" was not only on new drug and brain imaging but also on lifestyle as a cause, prevention and treatment.

Highlights of the conference included:

- Exploring the effect of avoiding stress and the positive effect of meditation on one's memory.

- The connection between lifelong psychological factors and the development of dementia.

- Social wellness, plus occupational and educational factors about probable culprits in the onset and progression of Alzheimer's disease. Nutritional factors as a predictor of risk in Alzheimer's disease.

- The therapeutic effects of herbal and vitamin supplements, especially Ginkgo biloba, Omega-3 and Vitamins C and E.

- Exercise and memory improvement.

Conferees who dealt with the complexities of Alzheimer's disease described their work as an art as well as a science, especially as they presented some of their more intriguing findings, theories and concepts that focused on lifestyles and their possible changes.

One excellent example was in the workshop of Dr. Dharma Singh Khalsa of the Alzheimer's Prevention Foundation, who said that he is now convinced more than ever that growing old doesn't go hand-in-hand with becoming senile. Dr. Khalsa referred to the many strategies that have been developed over the past decade to prevent brain deterioration in old age. Chief among these are the so-called "maintain your brain" tactics, which continue to demonstrate that an active mind is the key to preventing a later loss of brain function. The doctor spoke of how lifestyle changes, especially stress reduction, can lead to greater cognitive function in seniors. And in his seminal book *The Better Memory Kit, A Practical Guide to the Prevention and*

Reversal of Memory Loss, Including Alzheimer's, he tells of a very interesting encounter, which he calls *A Patient Regains Her Memory.* Linda, a forty-nine year-old writer and editor, attended one of Dr. Khalsa's seminars, and confessed that she believed she had early Alzheimer's, as her cognitive abilities had declined drastically and since there had been Alzheimer's in her family. She was having particular difficulty remembering and using words, which was deadly to her inasmuch as words were the tools of her trade. Dr. Khalsa at once put Linda on a program that included a nutritious diet, vitamin and stress-relieving supplements, memory-enhancing nutrients, a mind/body exercise program, and the hormone Pregnenolone, a memory stimulant. Within three months Linda reported that her speech difficulties, i.e. foggily groping to recall words and phrases, had greatly improved and that she was experiencing "good success" in remembering numbers and names. Dr. Khalsa states that Linda's level of response is by no means unusual. So there is good reason for optimism.

Indeed researchers have developed a number of studies showing a strong connection between cognitive and emotional health. In fact, stress can actually cause *structural changes* in the brain, so much so that a brain overwhelmed by stress can suffer major memory loss. In older people, acute stress is directly related to impairment of cognitive functioning. Families caring for a relative are under a great deal of stress, providing physical and emotional care and watching with horror the debilitating, horrific changes in their loved one. It can be very helpful for caregivers to use some tried-and-true stress reduction techniques including prayer, meditation, art, dance therapy, and exercise of various sorts, like stretching, *tai chi,* and yoga. It is also important for families to have respite care, with other persons frequently giving breaks to the primary caregiver(s). In addition, there are support groups wherein caregivers can openly and freely discuss their lives and emotions, and thus lessen stress through sharing and comparing. As they learn to better care for their own health through stress reduction, diet, and supplementation, they are innoculating themselves against Alzheimer's as well as developing strength and energy for the arduous tasks of care giving that lie ahead. Whatever methods are chosen, all are essential for care-givers, high-risk patients, and those with an already diminished brain capacity.

In addition to proper diet, exercise, and mental stimulation, physical and mental contact with others is a key part of prevention and treatment. Everyone benefits from hugs, touches, kind words, and someone with whom to share thoughts and feelings. A mental ping-pong game of ideas bouncing back and forth between two people keeps minds sharp. If someone knows an Alzheimer patient's personal history, it's even better because one can discuss the past. And understanding the past is therapeutic for improving the present and preparing a better future. One can repeat familiar family stories and humorous anecdotes. To be able to do all this, to keep up conversations even when the loved one cannot fully participate and ensure that proper foods and supplements are taken, is a rewarding but difficult job for anyone. It is for this reason that support groups and respite care services for families exist. Within the support groups for care givers, you will likely learn of the latest discoveries for coping with specific Alzheimer's symptoms and behaviors.

As an example, in one workshop of the convention, researchers from the Karolinska Institute in Stockholm presented findings on the relationship between early psychological factors and dementia. There is now a great deal of scientific interest in the "life-course" model for the risk of Alzheimer's disease and other dementias.

Data was gathered on pre-diagnosed patients for a six-year period to determine their lifestyles during childhood, adolescence, and adulthood. Factors such as education, socioeconomic status, work stress, and complexity of work, as well as leisure activities and social networks, were measured. The studies found that while a healthy psychological outlook is very important during all stages of life for preventing dementia, activities in later life, such as purpose, interests, hobbies, and social networking, are especially strong buffers against senility.

These ideas were reinforced by the work of the well-known neurophysiologist, Dr. Yaakov Stern of Columbia University, who also presented findings on the importance of lifestyle and other risk factors in the prevention of Alzheimer's disease. Dr. Stern has also done pioneering work in the treatment of Alzheimer's disease. He believes that symptoms of the disease may be offset even if the illness already exists, because of what he terms "cognitive reserve." This reserve is the sum total of early-life experiences including job-related and recreational activities, and whether we kept busy with our minds and hearts fully engaged, or let our minds stagnate and wither. Those who stayed mentally fit over the years seem to have an ability to delay or even halt the actual onset of pathology. Wherever the researchers were from, they arrived at similar conclusions. Another researcher, Caroline Herada of the University of Chicago, outlined the connection between the level of education (not necessarily formal) and occupational development and the incidence of dementia. The higher the level, the lower the incidence. This finding suggests that despite a biological or genetic predictor of the disease, simply using our brains can indeed affect whether we develop dementia or not. She suggests that certain mental activities in one's occupation may protect both the body and the mind. In all studies, the principles are the same for prevention, improvement of the condition, or reversal.

There is also important research underway that is concerned

with saving at-risk brain cells. Although even in Alzheimer's patients some cells are still healthy, some are already dead, and some are sick. If the sick ones can be cured, it is believed that mental function could be regained. Karen Ashe, a researcher and neurology professor at the University of Minnesota, is working on both the brain protein beta-amyloid, that harms brain cells, and on the recovery of cells that have been attacked by Alzheimer's, but are not yet dead. The Vice President of Medical and Scientific Affairs of the Alzheimer's Association , Dr. William Thies, believes that even if only a portion of the sick cells were rehabilitated, mental function could return. (Chicago Tribune, July 15, 2005) Since today's drugs treat only symptoms, family members have to make do with what is available: improving diet, exercise, reducing stress and, as much as possible, increasing mental stimulation.

Happily, research will continue, and we would be well-advised to keep up-to-date with developments concerning this disease because our knowledge is still in its infancy. Tests are now available to measure neurotransmitter capabilities. In order for lucid, concise thoughts to form, the transmitters must be clear and working. Other research is being conducted on ways to prevent excitotoxic changes— which cause nerve damage through excessive stimulation of the brain's excitatory amino acid (EAA) and increased formation of free radicals. Products being tested are those such as ibuprofen, Vitamin E, and Histamine Hz blockers like Tagamet. Still other studies are focusing on the prevention of plaque formation, as toxic plaque wedged between cells can cause neuronal death. Then there is also work on "super hormone" and antibody supple-ments to replace what our bodies lose with aging, such as DHEA and NGF. Also, studies are under way investigating the connection between a lack of hydrochloric stomach acid, which can prevent the absorption and circulation to the brain of key nutrients, and the onset of Alzheimer's. If necessary, hydrochloric acid can be taken orally as Glutamic Acid Hydrochloric. In all cases, nutritious food, supplements, physical and mental exercise, and stress reduction are certain to have a positive influence on both sufferer and family members.

It is one thing to be healthy and possess the ability to understand the components of creating a healthy mind and body; it is quite something else when one is stricken with a brain disease. The best assistance can usually be found in a special therapeutic environment dedicated to facilitating healthy living and avoiding any deviation from it. Creating this type of environment is more difficult when the patient lives at home, because social interaction often becomes very difficult. If the patient stays at home, the caregiver, usually a member of the same family, needs to understand the dynamics of trying to recreate a healthy mind. If not, the afflicted person cannot follow the principles and will not improve. In these cases the condition worsens, and conflicts become more bitter and destructive. On the other hand, if the caregiver understands the principles of mental stimulation and proper diet, not only is the patient helped, but the caregiver also benefits in his or her own preventative program.

The incredible difficulty of being an Alzheimer's caregiver is one reason this disease is so devastating for families. But when the caregiver believes in and follows the principles of mental stimulation and sound nutrition, as well as the other factors that I have outlined, positive feelings are transmitted both consciously and unconsciously, and the interaction becomes easier and more pleasant, fulfilling, and satisfying. The caregiver and the patient will begin to enjoy each other's presence. It is like the pleasure a piano teacher feels when a student learns and improves, or the satisfaction a trainer experiences when his or her pupil wins a swimming meet.

Now through the electronic media and books, more people

are learning of the benefits (and absolute human necessity!) of mental stimulation, as well as the immeasurable value of proper diet, exercise, and stress reduction for the prevention and treatment of so many degenerative diseases. So when family members hear the dreaded news of a loved one diagnosed with Alzheimer's, they will be more receptive to putting these principles into action. Learning that the sickness has been exacerbated, if not caused, by an unhealthy lifestyle, the family becomes willing to make changes for themselves and to help their family member to live with changes as well. This benefits not only the family but society at large, for today there is a legion of degenerative diseases, more than ever before. This is so, in part, because we are exposed to more and more poisonous chemicals in our food, water, and air; and we eat compulsively and self-destructively, consuming more fats, sugars, and empty calories than ever; and we engage in far less physical activity than prior generations. Everyone who understands this realizes that we cannot expect a drug to cure destructive living. We can only remove the causes and increase immunity with our own natural, personal changes.

There are other substances we ingest that may have an effect on Alzheimer's, both negative and positive. Anti-cholinergic medicines like Thorazine or Donnatal may help certain parts of the body, but can harm the brain's system of thought-transmission. On the other hand, products containing ibuprofen may delay the onset of Alzheimer's by reducing inflammation. Aspirin and Tylenol may not provide this same benefit. Inflammation is a known killer of brain cells. Cell inflammation and deposits of the amyloid protein produce toxic plaques found in Alzheimer's patients. Research is being done on other substances as well. There appears to be a causal relation between a lack of DHEA and Alzheimer's. DHEA-S protects nerve cells. These supplements, as well as Melatonin, a natural sleep-inducer, are being tried with Alzheimer's patients. Melatonin can help set the internal clock so that Alzheimer's patients don't react so strongly to the lack of light at sundown. Many Alzheimer's patients are affected by "Sundowner's Syndrome," causing them to aimlessly wander the house all night. Melatonin may lessen or prevent this. Still other experiments are under way on Nerve Growth Factor, or NGF—the prototype of polypeptides which help insure survival of sensory neurons in the nervous system—to learn if it can reverse cell shrinkage and thus aid in Alzheimer's prevention.

Great care must be exercised in prescribing treatment, for certain substances that are beneficial in small doses can be harmful in larger concentrations. One of these is zinc, an antioxidant which protects against Alzheimer's. It can also provide protection against strokes and heart disease. However, large doses can increase the formation of plaque in the brain, ironically causing Alzheimer's to accelerate. Iron is another such substance. The body needs iron for the blood, otherwise anemia results. But if too much is present, it can produce oxygen radicals that damage brain cells. Obviously a delicate and difficult balance must be struck.

Beyond what we ingest, our machines and their byproducts also affect our brains. It is now believed that electromagnetism is a factor in Alzheimer's. Electromagnetism emanates from cell phones, electric shavers, microwave ovens, hair dryers, etc., in fact from many standard accoutrements of contemporary Western societies. Exposure can disrupt cells of the immune system and adversely affect cerebral nerves. Knowledge of substances and products that impact the brain will help us promote our own health while at the same time helping protect loved ones. As the saying goes, forewarned is forearmed.

Truth and Knowledge

And so knowledge is power. It is a weapon with which to resist disease, to defend one's self and family. All we need to do is harness the knowledge to action.

The desire to learn the truth of existence, the yearning to know the reality behind a facade, to uncover the secrets of the gods as it were, is inherent in the human psyche. Deviation from truth damages health in all its dimensions, physical, mental, and moral. This has been recognized in some form among all cultures and civilizations. Only those who suffer mental deficiencies and aberrations—the sick—are exempt from this law. Perhaps that is why they fall ill. Truth relates to all dimensions of life. It is no accident that throughout history, religions including Judaism, Christianity, Buddhism, Hinduism, Islam, and the Tao, have emphasized the principle of truth as essential to wholeness, individuation, and good health. This principle is clearly mentioned repeatedly in the Old as well as the New Testaments.

In our time, science and medicine should search for healing truths of the natural world. However, we know that human beings have weaknesses, and that truth often conflicts with wishes and desires. Destructive desires enslave us, while following the truth frees us. In the most fundamental sense we are our own doctors. We must care for ourselves as no physician can, selecting the proper vitamins, pure water, and nourishing foods, and following life-paths that help our minds and bodies flourish. And when a loved one can no longer make rational choices, for better or worse we become that loved one's physician.

In dealing with the problem of Alzheimer's, it is sometimes difficult for doctors to transcend old mindsets and old habits. Many have been trained to handle unusual problems with a drug prescription. It is a simple way out, which most patients accept because of the awe with which doctors are regarded, and because it has always been that way. And, farmers do not normally come knocking on our doors to show us the antioxidizing benefits of broccoli and spinach. *We* must seek the changes which work best for us.

Of course, if our doctor says we have hypertension (high blood pressure), we have to decide if we want to take the medicine offered and/or supplements that help lower the pressure. But whatever we take, our blood pressure must be monitored regularly, because high blood pressure is dangerous to the brain. Any compromises of it, by heavy, prolonged stress, mini-strokes, or head trauma, are all high-risk factors for Alzheimer's. High blood pressure alone can have a deleterious effect on cognitive skills in later life. So we should strive to make whatever lifestyle changes we can to avoid dangers, *especially stress,* by which we are all constantly bombarded.

To return to our earlier example, if a condition of high blood pressure exists, dietary changes are in order; salt intake must be reduced and weight loss may be necessary. (For every ten pounds lost, blood pressure is reduced by 2.5 points.) Naturally, if we smoke, we must find ways to quit, and there are many. If we have high LDL cholesterol, we must find ways to lower it just as we have to increase our HDL levels when indicated. It is a good bet that a proper diet, along with the other factors outlined, will go a long way toward improving the condition. Again, we have to weigh the factors of medicines offered for prescription versus natural diet and supplementation, utilizing common sense and an instinctive feel for what works best in our bodies.

Studies are today being conducted to determine if cholesterol drugs, statins, have an effect on Alzheimer's prevention. In any case, higher levels of LDL cholesterol have been associated with cognitive impairment. Therefore it is imperative to lower them.

In all aspects of our health, we have to care for our bodies far more than we would even a fine-tuned race car, for even in the age of cloning, we can't trade them in for newer models.

There is another Alzheimer's indicator to watch for—our homocysteine level. The reader may well ask, *my what level?* Homocysteine is a tiny amino acid molecule, which, like cholesterol, is part of cellular structure. It is intended to be converted to an amino acid, with the help of Vitamin B-12 and folate. If we do not take in enough B-12, the homocysteine is not converted and a buildup ensues. Persons with high levels have twice the incidence of Alzheimer's as those with normal levels. At this writing, scientists are still working to uncover the exact connection. Taking B-12 and folic acid regularly lowers the homocysteine level. A fascinating study appearing in the inaugural issue of *Alzheimer's and Dementia: the Journal of the Alzheimer's Association,* showed that older adults whose diets were high in folate reduced their risk of Alzheimer's disease by half compared with those whose diets contained less than the Recommended Dietary Allowances (RDA). Folate is found in fish, soybeans, oranges, tomatoes, spinach, and grains, but is also contained in most vitamin supplements. Spinach is the one vegetable containing the most B-12, but a daily supplement is highly recommended as a matter of course. Says Maria Corrada, assistant professor of neurology at the University of California at Irvine, "Overall healthy diets seem to have an impact on limiting Alzheimer's disease risk."

Now that you have, hopefully, gained some new insight into Alzheimer's disease and some measures that can be taken to prevent, lessen, possibly even reverse its effects, you must decide how often and in what measure you employ them. Making life-changes should not be thought of in specific timeframes, like going on a two-week fad diet; good habits are worth cultivating forever, and will help you achieve a happier and fuller existence. Which, after all, is the sole purpose for enhancing our health.

Ultimately, our well-being depends upon our ability to free ourselves from the bondage of negative behaviors and to become strong enough and educated enough to follow the principles of nature, which are the truth of existence. All human problems are manifestations of deviation from truths. Naturally, it takes effort and discipline and time to create meaningful changes, but there is no real gain without a corresponding effort.

Chapter Nine
If It Happened for Some, It Can Happen for Others.

Following are summaries of a few Alzheimer's and dementia cases that have been immersed in a therapeutic environment, where notable improvements were realized. I include them because they clearly illustrate the basic principles of health that I learned from observing beneficial changes in patients and people over the course of time, and which I discuss in various ways throughout the pages of this book. Theoretical knowledge is important, but practical proof is required if theories are to be validated. The principles which guide healthy living—eating wholesome nutritious foods, breathing clean air and drinking pure water, getting regular physical exercise, reducing stress, obtaining sound sleep, stimulation of the mind and intellect, and moving about freely among all the elements of the natural world—seem so simple and obvious as to be not worth stating. And yet the direction of our lives over the past century has been in the exact opposite direction, toward the artificial, the mechanical, the unnatural, the polluted, and the toxic.

It requires an effort of mind and will to swim against the rising tide of misused technology with all its waste products that can harm as well as help our lives, and to unlearn many of the negative and destructive behaviors we adopt as a matter of course and take for granted. Yet if we are to survive and flourish as a species, we must make the effort and exercise good judgment always. The human mind is everything, and if we can but change our ways of thinking about our health, all good things will become possible.

Case One: Lou and Beverly

Lou Stevens was a seventy-eight year-old professional writer who had been married for forty-nine years to Beverly, his former high school sweetheart. Beverly was seventy-five.

She had always been strongly supportive of all aspects of Lou's writing; he had reached a point in his life where he could not work without her. Reflecting back, he realized there had been Alzheimer's symptoms in Beverly years earlier, which he had failed at the time to recognize. Yet they had not affected her supportive relationship with him. However, a year before the diagnosis of Alzheimer's was made, she began losing her ability to relate to him, and she began to become forgetful about important matters. The effect on Lou was shattering, beyond painful. It was as if the person who most mattered in his life had turned her back on him and repudiated him. He sought help from their physician, but when it was not forthcoming and serious conflicts and arguments arose with Beverly, in desperation he consulted a friend who told him of a resort-like health-care complex that specialized in caring for seniors, just built and opened on The Lake of Two Mountains near Montreal.

Insisting on entering the treatment center with Beverly to be close to her, Lou chose the traditional program, one reason for which was that the residence served very fine French cuisine. Lou decided at first to take two rooms, one for him and one for Beverly. Over the course of the next several months, he gradually became aware that those residents participating in Healthy Lifestyles programs looked, acted, and grew progressively stronger, more energetic, and more optimistic about life than those who did not participate. He opted to enter a specialized program himself, and enrolled Beverly in one appropriate to her condition. Both programs were based on physical exercise and sound nutritional principles: a vegetarian diet consisting predominantly of fresh fruits, green vegetables, nuts, whole grains, legumes, and for dessert a variety of fruit smoothies. Their diets were augmented with vitamins and mineral supplements.

Within six months Lou and Beverly slimmed down (both had been overweight), and his high blood pressure normalized. They participated together in yoga and therapeutic fitness classes conducted by Joseph Pilates (the revolutionary fitness guru and an old friend of mine), who visited the facility regularly from New York. In addition, Lou took part in group therapy sessions which greatly alleviated his fears for Beverly, thus dramatically reducing his own anxiety and stress.

At the same time, Lou, with relief and joy, began noticing major beneficial changes in his wife. She began behaving more normally, was calmer and less distant from him, and to a degree was able to resume her support of his various activities, especially as he grew to better understand her needs. After a year, they resumed living together in one suite, and a year after that, returned to their home and commenced completing a book they had begun earlier.

Both Lou and Beverly gained insight into her condition,

and modified their lifestyle according to what they had learned. They were then able to live together more lovingly and with much less friction.

Fortunately, Lou made the decision to adopt a healthy, therapeutic lifestyle in the nick of time. Had they begun earlier, perhaps Beverly's improvement might have been more significant. Yet it was significant enough to permit them to resume their lives together under the same roof, and that was a major victory for them both.

Case Two: Martin

Martin was seventy-two years old when his family and partners removed him from their business because he had become a destructive interference to the operation of their business. The consequences of what initially appeared to be careless and sometimes aggressive behavior became too serious to overlook or to overcome. He would shout and holler regularly because he could not remember what people said to him, or even what he demanded of them. Frightened and feeling powerless, it was almost as if a demon had taken possession of Martin. His family installed him in our program in the hope that he would live out the remainder of his days in some semblance of comfort and with a modicum of enjoyment.

At that time we did not specialize specifically in Alzheimer's because the disease was not as common as it is now, but the fundamentals of proper treatment were well in place. The program was multifaceted and available to all residents, regardless of which type of illness they suffered. We were able to observe clear improvement in all who participated.

By drastically improving Martin's diet, increasing his exercise, stimulating his interests and arousing his curiosity through group therapy and social interactions, he gradually but steadily became calmer, more relaxed, and improved his social skills. He even began volunteering to help other patients. After several months he expressed delight at living in such beautiful surroundings. At the end of a year, he had recovered to the extent that he was able to begin spending one day per week at his office, to the delight of his family. Still later he resumed many of his previous activities.

It is worth repeating: the earlier an Alzheimer's patient begins implementing lifestyle changes, the greater the chances of improving, and even reversing, many of the severest symptoms associated with the disease, especially in the area of memory and cognition.

Case Three: Terence and His Family

Also aged seventy-two was Terrance, whose wife, Edith, had died several years earlier. Heartbroken over the loss of his life-partner, Terrance had become a lost soul, steadily losing interest in the world around him, including his grown children and their families. Hurt and confused, they reacted negatively to his estrangement from them. They were not yet aware that he had been stricken with Alzheimer's. However, they were jolted into considering the possibility when they learned that he had nearly died in a kitchen fire he started by forgetting to turn the gas burners off and then falling asleep. They took him for a thorough hospital check-up and were given the sad news. Not having realized the extent of Terrance's deterioration, his children were sorry and felt guilty for misjudging his behavior, and at once placed him in our program.

Fortunately, the disease had been detected fairly early, and Terrance began progressive improvement. And as his condition improved, he became more and more aware of and interested in trying to help other members of his peer-group. When his family learned of these changes, they recalled with relief and joy that this had indeed been his way of life in the past. And they were further comforted by the fact that they had placed him in a comprehensive program quickly; early detection was as critical for their peace of mind and moral balance as it had been for Terrance's health and happiness.

Case Four: Herbert and Sally

Sally came to the program out of concern for what she described as her husband's failing memory, and fear that it may be Alzheimer's. "He seems to forget much more now. I have to plan for both of us…he doesn't comprehend as easily as before."

What was particularly upsetting to her was that he was "going through the same process of dementia as his sister did." Both Sally's mother and grandmother had suffered from Alzheimer's, and she was acutely aware of the disease having lived with it for so many years.

"He will ask about something, and we will discuss it, and then later on he will ask about the same thing we had previously spoken about. At other times he will be driving, and go down a one way street and not notice." Still other times he would run red lights, and get disoriented in areas he knew well. What was additionally upsetting to her was that Herbert had "exploded" at her twice in the past few months, and this was not like him.

Both Sally, 74, and Herbert, 78, spoke of a constant sense of anxiety in the pits of their stomachs.

Herbert did not speak of any memory difficulties, but rather his concern was his wife's anxiety and worrying. She would get terribly upset if he did not arrive home at the time she expected. However, what brought him to the program was his insomnia. He woke up between 3 and 4 a.m. every day, and couldn't get back to sleep. Over the past two years, his doctor had given him several different medications to help him sleep, but nothing helped. What he missed most was sleeping nestled alongside his wife. To wake up and lay next to her while she slept was lonely. Herbert spoke of the fact that the couple had been married for 52 years, and he was "crazy in love" with her, and missed doing everything with her.

The diagnostic history of the couple revealed that two years earlier, the couple had been involved in a car accident involving a young man running in front of their car in an attempt to kill himself. This event was eventually followed by Sally having a heart attack, from which she eventually recovered. The couple spoke of the fact that they had no religion or sense of spirituality in their life, and they felt that was missing.

Both Sally and Herbert entered the program which involved both individual and group sessions, in addition to the daily program and lifestyle modifications involving nutritional changes to their diet, exercise, and psychodynamic and cognitive behavioral interventions to address issues that came up in the course of the program. The couple immediately began learning and practicing techniques to lower the level of arousal of their sympathetic nervous system, which was contributing to the production of their symptoms. Through the psycho educational component of the program, both Sally and Herbert learned that they had been suffering from Post Traumatic Stress Syndrome, which resulted in maintaining them at a very high level of stress, and ultimately contributed to Sally's heart attack and Herbert's insomnia. Other longstanding family issues were effectively addressed, and Herbert was finally able to become a normal sleeper. Also he was delighted that he was now only waking up 1 to 2 times at night to go to the bathroom. Before beginning the program, he was getting up 5 to 6 times. He was no longer clenching his jaw, which was causing him pain. He also spoke about how much more patient he now felt.

Sally no longer suffered from her chronic anxiety in the pit of her stomach, and felt much more relaxed. Her difficulty with urinary incontinence improved significantly, and she felt much freer to be herself. The couple spoke about how much more relaxed they felt, and how they were able to laugh again. They expressed greater happiness and contentment, with Herbert commenting, "This is like a whole new life."

Sally spoke of the fact that Herbert was paying more attention to her. She also discussed the significant improvements in his memory and comprehension, and was so grateful for the improvement in their lives. The couple subsequently even planned a trip to Europe.

Case Five: Robert

Robert was a retired seventy-eight year old engineer; Stella, his wife, seventy-two, was a retired school teacher. Robert entered the program after becoming disoriented and lost a number of times, and was diagnosed with Alzheimer's. The family now realized that the disease symptoms had begun several years earlier, but that "no one wanted to admit it may be Alzheimer's." It was far too painful for them to face, and they attributed the symptoms to inconsequential lapses and the natural result of age.

All his life Robert had been a gentleman. He dressed in a suit and tie, was well-mannered and soft-spoken, and very kind and solicitous toward others. But over the past few years his personality had changed. Robert became less fastidious about his dress and personal grooming and hygiene, and his table manners deteriorated. Physically, he began to lose his hearing, along with his sense of smell. Unresponsive to others and forgetful of their names, his mood was most often one of irritation. He no longer arrived home on time or when expected.

Stella was extremely supportive of him in every way, but this did not prevent his hostility toward her; it only increased their mutual anguish. One resident later described him as "just plain ornery." No longer young, subject to her own infirmities, and emotionally distraught—being imprisoned beside a beloved husband who had become an abusive enemy was a 24-hour nightmare—Stella reached a point where she just could no longer cope with Robert and needed the assistance of a top-notch care facility with experts: therapists, nurses, dieticians, and staff skilled in handling Alzheimer's patients.

Slowly, gradually, Robert started to improve. He grew interested in a gardening project and eventually joined all the activities, and his social abilities rebounded. He started paying more attention to his manner of dress and began to enjoy coming to the dining room for meals. After a year, he looked more like his old self. But he was interested most of all in Stella, always waiting with excitement and anticipation for her to visit; their relationship was again becoming loving and supportive. He continued to expand his range of activities, made new friends, and expressed appreciation for being in the "retirement home." Each day he complimented the meal preparation and looked forward to daily events.

Case Six: Linda

A retired pathologist, Linda was a seventy-four year-old widow who lived alone. Her husband, a cardiologist, had died a year earlier. Linda walked very slowly, shuffling and mostly looking down at the ground.

She began her therapeutic sessions by listing the symptoms which troubled her. She spoke at length of memory problems, a cause of great anxiety and concern, and mentioned that her deceased mother had had Alzheimer's. She was tearful and continually wiped her nose with a tissue she kept tucked under her sleeve. No longer able to drive because of the physical pain of clambering in and out of her car, she was also experiencing depression. Her sleep was constantly interrupted by bathroom trips, and when she awoke in the morning she was tired and in pain. She also suffered from shortness of breath, and aching joints. She feared she had Parkinson's disease. Other feelings included guilt, sadness, distrust, resentment, helplessness, isolation, and a lack of control. She complained of estrangement from her son. She described a sense of *slowness*, a feeling that life had ceased moving, and that it seemed empty and devoid of meaning. Being prone to procrastination, she had difficulty making decisions, had lost her sense of humor and creativity, and no longer took any interest in her appearance.

When asked about her diet, she said that as a physician she maintained a busy schedule but believed she ate efficiently and obtained all necessary nutrients. She pointed out that she regularly took in vegetables, but did so by exclusively drinking "V-8" vegetable juice! She felt that her meals were "balanced" because they contained a meat, vegetable, and potato portion: she ate frozen dinners in front of the television. Linda was oblivious to how damaging all this processed food was: calorie-dense and deficient in nutritional value, laced with sodium, sugar, artificial ingredients, high-fat, and toxic chemicals.

Still grief-stricken, she spoke of how much she missed her husband, and of the shock and the huge void his death (he had died from a massive heart attack) had left. In truth, they had both lived unhealthily. They were strictly sedentary, taking no exercise whatever, and spent their hours together at home reading or sitting in front of the fireplace. Neither of them had any religious or spiritual beliefs.

The test results for Parkinson's came back negative but were indicative of Alzheimer's. Unsurprisingly, in addition to her other maladies, Linda had high blood pressure.

In so fragile and debilitated a state, the single most significant factor in arresting, or even improving, her condition would be a renewed sense of purpose and a restoration of hope. But first it would be necessary to wean her away from her deadly diet in order to build up her immunity. "They never taught us about diet in medical school," she confessed.

Over the course of the next several months, she was fed a wholesome, balanced diet which completely eliminated processed foods. Therapeutic exercises combined with group therapy and education on improving overall physiological and psychological health resulted in the beginnings of a new attitude and outlook, a feeling that life was not hopeless and that she was by no means helpless. She adopted a daily walking regimen and used her growing ability to cover longer distances as a marker of improvement. She volunteered for a literacy program and helped others to learn to read. She also began to engage the chaplain in religious and philosophical discourses, which turned out to be regular events which she greatly enjoyed and always looked forward to.

During group therapy sessions she learned non-pharmacological methods of managing stress and overcoming depression, in addition to ways of decreasing pain and hypertension through a combination of proper diet, exercise, breathing, and relaxation techniques. Education regarding the workings of human memory and factors which affect it for good or bad greatly lessened her anxiety and, by relaxing her, helped to improve her overall cognitive functioning, especially her memory.

As Linda became more and more conscious of correct eating, her physical infirmities underwent a marked change for the better, which in turn sparked an improvement in her *mental* health and outlook. Morning fatigue disappeared and she no longer complained of back pain. Most heartening was that she was not tormented by memory loss. "It's just not an issue anymore," she exulted. "I have so much energy and am so busy that I don't have time to worry." Moreover, she was no longer awakening five to six times per night to go to the toilet, but merely once or twice. She was even able to discontinue pain medication for her arthritis.

Over the course of the next year, Linda became progressively more involved and in charge of her own health management and recovery. She shed the old feelings of isolation and helplessness and became an advocate for other patients on behalf of powerful lifestyle changes, in particular the importance of adding a fulfilling spiritual and metaphysical dimension to life.

Case Seven: My Own Story—Dr. Anbar

An incurable disease is one which, while the cause exists, the human body cannot heal on its own, and which conventional medicine cannot cure because it lacks a pharmaceutical drug to do so. But does that really mean it is incurable?

Since I was a child I have believed that all ailments are ultimately curable, and my mind was always open to any and all possibilities. The trick lies in uncovering the correct approach. In those days I was quite sickly and could not participate in sports and games at school. I suffered constant indigestion and a stomach ulcer and had frequent colds which kept me in bed for periods of time. According to my physician, I also had a cardiac problem and I was forbidden from participating in sports.

I was taken to see the best conventional physicians, but they could offer no solutions. Then at age fourteen and on my own, I was lucky enough to come across a doctor who had cured his own numerous ailments strictly through a vegetarian diet and the development of healthful eating habits. Surprised by so simple a precept—I probably expected to hear some grandiose medical formulation—but deciding to follow his example and formula, I recovered completely within six months and commenced playing sports including martial arts, exceeding many of my peers within a year's time. Everyone perceived this as a great miracle (which it was, but for different reasons than they supposed) and since then I have devoted my life to Health.

I learned a crucial truth at that young age, and it has remained with me to this day: *the key to health and longevity is in the mind, because the mind controls all behavior.* I pursued my studies over the years with the mind-body link uppermost in my thoughts, and concentrated on taking an eclectic, holistic approach toward curative possibilities, however unusual they might seem and in whatever circumstances they might be found. While my studies were conventional for the most part, my natural inclination has always been to try to look at life in its totality—physical, psychological, and spiritual—rather than in its individual isolated components. If I heard of any one who had recovered from a supposedly incurable disease, my reaction was not that it was impossible and that the medical facts must have been wrong; rather I was curious and interested to know all the details to find out how and why an original cure had been effected.

In the course of my life I have observed that the overwhelming majority of those who recovered from so-called incurable diseases did so by exchanging unhealthy lifestyles for healthy ones. They accomplished this primarily by means of nutrition, but also by changes in outlook and through physical exercise which, coupled with proper diet, increased immunity, strength and resistance to infection. As with the bodily systems they affect, none of these methods work perfectly in isolation; they are interrelated and inextricably linked.

Interestingly, I have witnessed other types of surprise recoveries, that is, recoveries made outside the bounds of traditional Western medicine with the aid of "healers." Personally I had never been able to believe in the existence of true healers, in the laying on of hands, or in the healing propensities of yogis, shaman, fakirs, llamas, and the like. That is, until one day when I arrived in Cuernavaca, Mexico, and met an American woman who changed my mind about such things.

One year earlier she had been quite ill. She had been hospitalized in Mexico but could not be cured. She returned home to a Los Angeles hospital, but nothing could be done. Feeling trapped and desperate, she went back to Cuernavaca to meet a friend who had told her of a healer in Mexico City who worked wonders. She decided to see him. After just a few sessions with him, she made a full and complete recovery.

Difficult as it was to believe in what had happened, I asked for and received an introduction to the healer. His name was Eriberto and he worked with groups of the sick. He called the work "cleansing." He never touched patients physically, preferring to work only with their auras, which it is said all people possess. I sat in with a group and watched him work. Toward the end of the session, to my utter astonishment, he turned to me and stunned me by telling me things about myself he could not possibly have known or have ever heard. It was immediately clear that he had a very special sensitivity and insight. But even more impressive were the stories his patients told about him.

I met a famous stage-actress who told of being diagnosed for cancer while in Mexico, and who then went to Houston for a second opinion and additional examination. She spent several days there and the cancer was confirmed. It was recommended that she undergo surgery immediately. At that point a friend told her about Eriberto, and she decided to see him before submitting to the operation. After only a few visits she began to feel better; her symptoms started to diminish. She returned to Houston to recheck the diagnosis and was informed she no longer had cancer!

My own numerous observations of Eriberto at work confirmed this: while he worked with a person, he was transformed, a love and healing energy flew out of him and suffused and encompassed the individual. So profound was this energy that even an objective observer could feel, and even see, the emanations.

I had another very unusual experience, this time in Europe. While visiting a Thalaso therapy (ocean water therapy) center in Germany, I met a man who had suffered from acute arthritis but who had been cured completely by a healer near Stockholm, Sweden. Curious and highly interested, I obtained her phone number and made an appointment to see her.

A handsome woman in her early seventies, in excellent physical condition, she ran a small institute for those afflicted with severe arthritis. When I arrived at her office she showed me pictures of herself from a time past when arthritis nearly crippled her; parts of her body had been totally deformed. She cured herself by herself, and thereafter dedicated her life to curing others. Her work, wildly successful decades before research confirmed her methods, consisted of two parts. Part one was to place patients on a strict cleansing diet of fruits and vegetables. Part two was *touching* the affected body areas with an incredibly energizing warmth and love, which she was somehow able to project. It was a strange and wonderful sight I shall never forget.

There is now solid evidence—recent researches indicating that such methods are not nearly as exotic or outlandish as they may at first appear. Researchers have shown that eating brightly colored fruits and vegetables can help lower the risk of developing rheumatoid arthritis by increasing immunity and fighting inflammation. With only a modest increase in antioxidants from the raw fruits and vegetables the risk of developing inflammatory arthritis is being diminished. For it has long been known that oxidation (and its harmful byproduct, free radicals) plays a role in joint damage. The researchers believe that antioxidants suppress inflammation throughout the body by destroying free radicals.

These unorthodox healing methods are not yet considered scientific in the strict sense because extensive university studies and experiments have not yet been conducted in these areas, although this is changing. On the other hand, the facts of what I and many others have witnessed are indisputable. All those sick folks who flocked to Eriberto had incurable diseases. They turned to him because conventional medicine was of no avail; and all of them say they have fully recovered as a result of his efforts. To quote William Shakespeare, "There are more things between heaven and earth, Horatio, than are dreamt of in your philosophy."

Afterword
Now is a Time for Real Action—
Relaxation

The relaxation response is the opposite physical and mental condition to the stress response. It is a condition characterized by a lowered metabolic rate and a calm state of mind.

"We can lessen the effects of stressful thoughts through the repetition of a prayer, word, sound, phrase, or muscular activity. When the relaxation response is elicited, the harmful effects of norepinephrine are counteracted. In so doing, we tap into billions of years of healing capacities."

—Dr. Herbert Benson, Harvard Medical School

There she stands, smiling, tall and erect, physically vibrant, a twinkle in her eye, the woman who cared for you when you were ill, who taught you to read, to cook, to sing, to look both ways before crossing the street. She is your mother.

These days, she is busy exercising at the health club, playing bridge with her group, seeing a new film at the multiplex, or at the health store picking up fresh organic produce for her latest recipes. You no longer need to worry about her mind; her memory is as sharp as your own. She is happy and enjoys telling a good joke every now and then. She was previously diagnosed with Alzheimer's, and her improvement is astonishing. If it happened for her, it can happen for others.

Now that you know there are powerful ways to help your loved one and that there are preventions available for yourself, you must relax as much as possible and realize that any problem, including a degenerative health problem, is also a golden opportunity to improve: to change bad habits into good ones, and to lead a long, vigorous, healthy, fulfilling life. Today, with a better understanding of the principles of nature, of potent natural multidimensional treatment methods at our disposal, the body afflicted with Alzheimer's can be viewed more like a neglected car, in need of a tune-up and oil change to ensure optimum performance. Families no longer need to feel guilty and helpless while watching relatives slip into dementia; we can *choose* to adopt healthful, restorative measures in diet and exercise, and retention of the proper therapeutic environment to nurture loved ones. In deciding to improve your dietary habits and incorporate stress-reducing activities, as well as maintaining a variety of interests and choosing an active lifestyle, it is comforting to know that new medical treatments are being researched and developed that hold out hope to hasten recovery.

We are on the cusp of an exciting new age in the prevention and treatment of Alzheimer's, for scientific medicine is at long last beginning to view patients holistically. We are something more than an agglomeration of cells and chemical processes; rather, we are whole persons with intertwining physical, spiritual, and psychological selves. This is something that Eastern philosophy with its emphasis on the mind/body link has understood for millennia, as embodied in the lives of the Hunza. Whether for yourself or for your loved one, after listening to the advice of trusted doctors, psychologists or counselors, in the end you alone must decide how best to proceed. But no matter what medicines or treatments may emerge in the future, healthy and nutritious foods, exercise, stress-management, a healthy emotional and spiritual life, in short, living healthily—it truly *is* the best medicine—and will always be on the cutting edge of healing science. It is the foundation upon which any new discoveries must be built. Following is a brief summary of some emerging helpful medicinal possibilities:

1. The drug Alzehemed is being tested to learn if it removes from the body the toxic protein beta amyloid, which can clump together to form brain-plaque. Alzehemed may bind the beta strands and filter it from the body.

2. A blood protein product called IVIg is being tested to determine if it can be an effective antibody against beta amyloid. It could especially benefit older persons, whose bodies produce less of these natural antibodies than do those of younger people.

3. Intravenous immunoglobulin is under study to determine if it can increase antibodies. In trials, patients were found to be more alert and articulate.

3. Gamma secretase, an enzyme, blocks A-beta. However, this enzyme also blocks proteins that protect the brain. Scientists are working on a drug that would create a weak gamma secretase that would block only the A-beta.

4. Leuprolide, a hormone used in treating prostate cancer, may also be helpful in treating Alzheimer's.

5. Scientists are currently at work on a nasal vaccine which would reduce brain-plaque typically seen in Alzheimer's sufferers. So far, the vaccine has been tested on mice. "It works in mice," says Howard Weiner, M.D., co-director of the Center for Neurological Diseases at Harvard Medical School. "The next step is to see whether it's safe in humans and then we can test to see how efficacious it is." The vaccine mixes an FDA-approved multiple sclerosis drug and an additional substance that helps the vaccine stimulate immunity. The nasal vaccination could be given as a spray or as drops.

Clearly all of this research and testing takes time that can never replace what we can do immediately, which is to adopt a *proactive approach* to healing, by taking the preventive measures I have outlined and discussed throughout the pages of this book. Certainly we live in a society which breeds stress. All of us must learn to turn off our anger switches and tone down our wild emotional reactions to the grind and pressures of simple daily living: fury over the traffic and congestion and the endless lines and crowds, outrage at the sloppy service and exorbitant prices we encounter, at the rudeness, selfishness, discourtesy, and rancor of our fellow man, at the incessant noise, the constant overwhelming din, at the smog, the pollution, and the ten thousand other irritants and stress-producers that assault us in the course of our regular routines. We simply cannot afford to allow that which is beyond our control to destroy our minds and bodies, to eat us alive, to devour us from the inside out.

There are some simple but effective countermeasures we

can take: we can do the things human beings have always done, as were done in ancient times by shepherds and other healthy, hearty, agrarian folk. We can sing softly and we can dance and we can listen to music, which soothes the savage beast. We can contemplate a sunrise, watch a puppy frolic or a kitten purr, walk in the woods or read a poem. We can be moved by music, listen to waves lapping a shoreline; we can ponder a piece of inspiring art. We can read a book and then compare it to the film; we can sit in the soothing water of a warm tub even when we do not need a bath. Despite contemporary life's massive pressures, there are places and things we can escape to, and we should go to them as frequently as we must and as often as we can.

Of course, some stress is natural and normal, a part of life, of human existence. Our bodies and minds will react violently to a child in a burning building, or to a Bengal tiger charging toward us. That would obviously not be the time to try our new relaxation techniques; we would want our adrenaline pumping (our legs, too!) and our thoughts racing. Even a fleeting stress causes chemical changes in the brain, so imagine the havoc a prolonged stress of months or years will wreak. When under stress, the body produces cortisol which suppresses the immune system, lowering resistance to disease. Hans Selye and Herbert Benson have defined excessive and unhealthy stress as an inability to cope with the stress-inducer, resulting in a feeling of inadequacy and depression. But they also point out that we must never forget that it is not so much a given situation that produces destructive stress, as how we react and respond to particular conditions. Exercise is a natural stress-buster, as is a balanced diet that provides adequate energy and constantly replenishes lost nutrients, and which helps control blood pressure and stabilize blood-sugar levels. Joe Weider, founder of the

multimillion   dollar   bodybuilding/nutritional/publishing
empire Weider Enterprises (which includes the popular *Men's
Health, Shape,* and *Muscle and Fitness* magazines), is in his late
eighties and has never been sick with a major illness in his life
because he has combined vigorous fitness activity with nutri-
tionally sound eating principles ever since he was a teenager.

When a new day dawns, view it as an opportunity to
improve body, mind, and soul. Try to contribute something
positive, no matter how simple or small, to your life and the
lives of others. Having a plan of sorts helps, but learning to
deal calmly and effectively with what happens if the plan goes
awry is one of the keys to real relaxation. If you refuse to
become discouraged and can develop an ability to take advantage of unexpected changes and circumstances, you will benefit not only your blood pressure but your immune system,
your endocrine system, and your cardiovascular system. Yet
don't make the mistake of attempting to schedule and regi-
ment every waking moment of every waking hour. Take rest-
breaks when you can. Get into the habit of meditating. When
you return from the break, you'll be refreshed and better able
to tackle the tasks that await, more prepared to handle and
overcome the inevitable difficulties and stresses. If you can
learn to do these things, and you can, the results will be astonishing. You will empower yourself and decide how to react to
the people you meet and the situations you confront. You'll
certainly be more relaxed, and you'll be well on your way to a
healthier brain function and a happier, longer life. You will
have a stronger immunity to all degenerative illnesses, including Alzheimer's.

Remember: Life and health are based on principles— the
Laws of Nature. We must know, respect and follow them. If
you want to help in recovering from Alzheimer's, the best thing

to do for the victim is to immerse him or her into a therapeutic environment that fully facilitates following the Laws of Nature with love and compassion, and prevents as much as possible any deviation from these laws.

Our lives depend on the choices we make. We must all choose wisely.

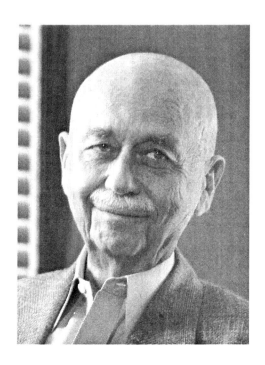

About the Author

Abraham, Isaac Anbar, B.A., M.A., M.S., Sc.D., C.A.S.Ed., was educated at the American University Beirut, the Hebrew University Jerusalem, Calvin Coolidge College, Simmons College, and Harvard University.

Dr. Anbar has been a pioneer in the healthcare, hospital, residential and institutional field for over 50 years. Beginning his career in 1953 as an Associate Professor of Psychiatry at McGill University, he subsequently founded and operated Canada's largest and most prestigious private chain of therapeutic residential facilities for children, adolescents and adults suffering from mental and neurological disabilities – collectively known as the Anbar Institutes, in addition to facilities for the elderly, providing life-span care unequaled in the industry.

Many of Dr. Anbar's innovations in congregate, skilled nursing and hospital and healthcare management have been used as models for facilities in the United States, Canada and abroad. Succeeding expansion of the Anbar organization led to developments in the United States, the Middle East and Mexico. In the area of cardiovascular health, in the 1960's, the organization was the first to introduce the concept of cardiovascular rehabilitation in the Midwest U.S., and installed cardiac rehabilitation units in major medical centers and hospitals. The organization's research and development projects resulted in the development of technologies for cardiovascular intervention, software development for hospital administration and rehabilitation devices. For the major health care organization in Israel, Kupat Cholim owned by the Labour Party, the Anbar organization developed the healthcare industry's largest multi-phasic medical diagnostic center in the world specializing in early detection and intervention, currently diagnosing over 55,000 patients per month. At the invitation of various families of patients and health care professionals in Mexico, the first Anbar-affiliated Institute was opened in Mexico City in 1970, as a resource for the care of children and adolescents suffering from developmental and neurological conditions, as well as seniors suffering from chronic and degenerative diseases. In Canada, the Anbar Institutes were acquired by the government of Quebec to form part of the province's healthcare system.

Currently, Dr. Anbar continues to concentrate on searching for and developing the best solutions for the prevention and treatment of Alzheimer's and other degenerative diseases, as well as the underlying factors in preserving health and longevity.

Bibliography

Alzheimer's Activities: Hundreds of Activities for Men and Women with Alzheimer's Disease and Related Disorders, by B.J. Fitzray. Rayve Productions, 2001. 288 pages.

Alzheimer's Disease by Frena Gray-Davidson. Judy Piatkus Publisher Ltd, 1999.

Alzheimer's Disease, by Elwood Cohen. Keats Publishing, 1999. 253 pages.

Alzheimer's Disease, by Paul D. Dash and Nicole Villemarette-Pittman. Demos Medical Publishing, 2005. 156 pages.

Beating Alzheimer's by Tom Warren. Avery, 1991. 240 pages.

Brain Allergies; The Psychonutrient Connection by William H. Philpot, MD and Dwight K. Kalita, PhD. McGraw-Hill, 2000. 256 pages.

Brain Longevity, by Dr. Dharma Singh Khalsa. Warner Books, 1997, 440 pages.

Eat To Live, by Dr. Joel Fuhrman. Little, Brown, 2003. 280 pages.

Fight Alzheimer's Naturally, by Cathy Picoulin. Crown Publishing, 1998. 192 pages.

Food As Medicine by Dharma Singh Khalsa, MD. Atria, 2002. 368 pages

Food: Your Miracle Medicine, by Jean Cooper. Harper Paperbacks, 1994. 560 pages.

Healing the Soul in the Age of the Brain by Elio Frattaroli. Penguin Books, 2002. 464 pages.

Mayo Clinic on Alzheimer's Disease, by Mayo Clinic (Corporate Author), Ronald C. Petersen (Editor). Kensington Publishing Corporation, 2002. 192 pages.

New Hope for People with Alzheimer's and Their Caregivers by Porter Shimer. Three Rivers Press, 2002. 304 pages.

Power Over Stress by Kenford Nedd, MD. QP press, 2004. 224 pages.

Prescription for Nutritional Healing by James F. Balch, MD & Phyllis A. Balch, CNC. Avery, 2000. 784 pages.

The 36-Hour Day: A Family Guide to Caring for Persons with Alzheimer's disease, Related Dementing Illnesses, and Memory Loss in Later Life, by Nancy L. Mace and Peter V. Rabins. Warner Books, 2001. 512 pages.

The Better Memory Kit, A Practical Guide to the Prevention and Reversal of Memory Loss, Including Alzheimer's, by Dr. Dharma Singh Khalsa. CDs, memory cards, 2004.

The Biology of Belief, by Bruce Lipton, Ph.D. Mountain of Love/Elite Books, 2005. 210 pages.

The Everyday Alzheimer's Book by Carolyn Dean, MD. Adams Media Corporation, 2004. 289 pages.

The Inflammation Cure: How to Combat the Hidden Factor behind Heart Disease, Arthritis, Asthma, Diabetes, Alzheimer's Disease, Osteoporosis, and Other Diseases of Aging, by William Joel Meggs and Carol Srec. NTC Publishing, 2003. 238 pages.

The Memory Cure by Majid Fotuhi, MD, PhD. McGraw-Hill, 2004. 256 pages.

The pH Miracle, by Robert O. Young, Ph.D., and Shelley Redford Young. Time Warner Book Group, 2003. 340 pages.

The Power of the Mind to Heal by Joan Borysenko, PhD and Miroslav Borysenko, PhD. Hay House, 1995. 240 pages.

The Psychological Bulletin, a Publication of the American Psychological Association. Sergerstrom study published July, 2005.

Who Gets Sick? by Blair Justice, PhD. Peak Press, 2000. 464 pages.

Index